BASIC BONE RADIOLOGY

BASIC BONE RADIOLOGY

Harry J. Griffiths, M.D.

Associate Professor of Radiology and Orthopedics
Department of Diagnostic Radiology
The University of Rochester Medical Center
Rochester, New York

APPLETON-CENTURY-CROFTS/New York

81 82 83 84 85/10 9 8 7 6 5 4 3 2 1

Prentice-Hall International, Inc., London
Prentice-Hall of Australia, Pty. Ltd., Sydney
Prentice-Hall of India Private Limited, New Delhi
Prentice-Hall of Japan, Inc., Tokyo
Prentice-Hall of Southeast Asia (Pte.) Ltd., Singapore
Whitehall Books Ltd., Wellington, New Zealand

Library of Congress Cataloging in Publication Data

Griffiths, Harry J
   Basic bone radiology.

    Includes index.
    1. Bones—Radiography. I. Title. [DNLM:
1. Bone and bones—Radiography. WE225 G855b]
RC930.5.G74   616.7'107572   80-21741
ISBN 0-8385-0535-X

Text design: Holly A. Reid
Cover design: Janet Koenig

To P.A.M.

the perpetual student
—with affection and thanks

Contents

Preface

This text is based both on a short introductory course given to successive fourth-year medical students as well as on introductory lectures on bone radiology which the author has given to orthopedic residents. The book has been expanded to include some important but rarer conditions even though it is meant solely as an "introduction to bone radiology."

The book begins with an introductory chapter, which defines many of the commonly used terms. There is also a brief description of the cellular structure and formation of bone, as well as an overview of the radiographic appearance of many common skeletal conditions given in tabular form. The subsequent six chapters cover the most important bone diseases with respect to congenital, traumatic, infective and metabolic conditions, arthritis, and tumors. Since, in the author's opinion, there is no adequate outline of common bone tumors available, Chapter 7 is slightly longer than is probably appropriate for an introductory text. The information in this chapter is presented in a telegraphic manner. Chapter 8 covers specialized radiographic procedures that are relevent to the skeleton and Chapter 9 covers a potpourri of diseases and situations that are difficult to find in many more extensive books on bone disease.

The concept of this book is to provide a basic text on bone radiology to residents in either radiology or in orthopedics and to fourth-year medical students. The text has been deliberately kept short, the tables and diagrams have been used to enhance it where useful. Based on ten years of teaching experience, the illustrations have been selected not only to illustrate the text but also very often to amplify it, thus making sense of the decision to put the text first, followed by the illustrations.

As Seneca said: "Even while they teach, men learn." I have enjoyed both teaching and learning and I trust you learn as much as I have from putting this text together.

Acknowledgments

I would like to thank many of my former students and residents who not only stimulated me to teach "An Introduction to Bone Radiology" but also suggested that my material should be published in a more palpable form. I would also like to thank those people who helped prepare the manuscript: particularly Alyce Norder who did all the initial typing and drew the diagrams and Belinda DeLibero who remained unfailingly cheerful while typing the final manuscript and proofs. The illustrations have been gleaned from many sources over the years and although the majority of the patients are my own, I would like to thank the Radiology Staff of Children's Hospital in Boston (particularly Thorne Griscom, M.D. and Robert Wilkinson, M.D.) for the use of some of the pediatric cases. I would also like to thank Stanley Bohrer, M.D. for examples of the more unusual infections. I must apologize to those people whose cases are included and whom I have inadvertently not acknowledged. Finally I would like to thank both Doreen Berne and Holly Reid of Appleton-Century-Crofts for being so supportive and helpful while the book was in its final stages.

Fairport, New York, July 1980

BASIC BONE RADIOLOGY

ONE

Introduction

Since this book is an introduction to the radiology of skeletal disease, there is no necessity to go into bone morphology in any detail. The reader interested in more detailed information is referred either to the standard texts or to a number of more specialized books. (See the references at the end of this chapter.)

Before approaching the various specific disease entities that are discussed in subsequent chapters, an introduction to some commonly used terms and their meaning is appropriate:

THE PHYSEAL (OR EPIPHYSEAL) PLATE.   This consists of five layers of progressively maturing bone: the resting zone, the zone of proliferation, the zone of hypertrophy, the zone of calcification, and finally the zone of ossification (Fig. 1-1). Bone formation occurs on both sides of the plate to form the *epiphysis* at the end of the bone and the *metaphysis* which is the major growing part of the shaft of the long bone. The physeal plate is lucent radiographically.

THE EPIPHYSIS (OR SECONDARY GROWTH CENTER).   This is at the end of a long bone and is formed from within a cartilaginous analogue. When fully matured the epiphysis becomes fused to the metaphysis as the involution of the physeal plate occurs. This can be seen at various ages from 4 up to 21 depending on which epiphysis is concerned. Strictly speaking, the epiphysis ceases to exist once this fusion and involution of the physeal plate has occurred.

THE METAPHYSIS.   This is the growing part of a long bone and lies between the physeal plate and the *diaphysis.* Two processes are involved in bone modeling: One is *bone growth* which occurs at the physeal plate and into the metaphysis; the other is *tubulation* which occurs as a result of periosteal resorption of bone in the metaphyseal region (Fig. 1-2). Tubulation may fail due to certain situations such as absence of normal periosteal osteoclasis (as is seen in osteopetrosis) or an overgrowth of the intramedullary components (such as is seen in Gaucher's disease), whereupon the metaphyseal ends of the long bones flare out. This is said to resemble an Erlenmeyer flask if it is seen in the lower femur (Fig. 1-2B, Table 1-1). Tubulation becomes exaggerated in certain other conditions where there is excessive periosteal osteoclasis, and this apparent thinning of the metaphyses occurs in paralysis, poliomyelitis, cerebral palsy, and disuse osteoporosis in children where long thin "gracile bones" can be seen (Fig. 1-2C).

Table 1-1

Erlenmeyer Flask Deformity
Osteopetrosis
Metaphyseal dysplasias including craniometaphyseal dysplasia, achondroplasia, Pyle's disease
Biliary atresia
Gaucher's disease
Hypophosphatasia
Thalassemia
Lead intoxication
Healing rickets or scurvy
Multiple enchondromas (Ollier's disease) or multiple osteochondromas

THE DIAPHYSIS.   This is the central part of the shaft of a long bone and embryologically actually represents the *primary growth center.* Although apparently a hollowed out cortical tube after the age of 2 or so, up to that time a complex series of processes have been occurring in the diaphysis including endosteal osteoclasis which produces the marrow cavity. If this process fails for any reason, such as occurs in osteopetrosis where there is an almost total failure of osteoclasis both endosteally and periosteally, no marrow cavity is formed and the child eventually dies of anemia (Fig. 1-3).

There are three basic bone cells: (1) the *osteoblast,* which forms bone, (2) the *osteoclast,* which resorbs bone, and (3) the *osteocyte,* which is the resting cell found mainly within trabeculae and in the Haversian canals of cortical bone. Until recently, these three cells were thought to be separate offshots of a primordial mesenchymal progenitor cell, however, a number of researchers have recently demonstrated an interrelationship between them. The multinucleated osteoclast is apparently able to disintegrate into uninuclear osteoblasts or even into a "resting" osteocyte. This process appears to be stimulated by certain biochemical, hormonal, and even structural influences. The osteocyte itself can become stimulated under certain circumstances to resorb bone (*osteocytic osteoclasis*). This process may actually be demonstrated radiographically using high resolution film or magnification studies. It is known as "intracortical tunneling" and is due to osteocytic widening of the Haversian systems. It can be seen in hyperparathyroidism (both primary and secondary), osteomalacia, thyrotoxicosis, and in disuse states (such as paralysis and disuse osteoporosis).

These bone cells are on a supporting base known as the *osteoid*, which is a term referring to osseous tissue prior to calcification. Osteoid may be mineralized or unmineralized and is itself based on a collagen matrix which has fibrous tissue and cartilaginous components. Naturally various things can go wrong at any stage of bone formation with the collagen matrix itself (leading to osteogenesis imperfecta), to the fibrous base (leading to fibrous dysplasia), or to the cartilaginous tissue (probably accounting for the increased incidence of benign and malignant cartilaginous tumors seen in the pelvis, shoulder girdle, and ribs). The process of mineralization of osteoid requires the presence of adequate amounts of both calcium and vitamin D as well as the correct balance of the various hormones involved in bone formation, particularly the parathyroid hormone, an excess of which leads to hyperparathyroidism or *osteitis fibrosa et cystica* (see Chap. 5).

PRIMARY TRABECULAE.   These are the weight-bearing trabeculae and follow the lines of stress. They are particularly well seen in the pelvis, femoral necks, and vertebral bodies.

SECONDARY TRABECULAE.   These are the smaller transverse and oblique trabeculae which are often difficult to appreciate on conventional radiographs. In osteoporosis, the secondary trabeculae are resorbed first leading to apparent accentuation of the primary trabeculae and also of the end plates in the vertebral bodies.

CORTICAL BONE.   This term refers to the tubular structures of the long bones. Measurements of cortical bone width can be used for assessing bone mineral, particularly referring to the Metacarpal Index which is the ratio of cortical thickness to the whole width of the second metacarpal at its midpoint. This should be about 45 percent in normal people and may be as low as 10 percent in patients with severe osteoporosis.

CANCELLOUS BONE.   This accounts for the remainder of the skeletal bone and particularly the vertebral bodies; the flat bones such as the pelvis, ribs, and scapulae; and the metaphyseal ends of the long bones. Theoretically, loss of bone mineral occurs equally throughout the skeleton and thus simultaneously in both cancellous and cortical bone. Since cancellous bone accounts for about 80 percent of our skeletal weight, however, it is obvious that minute changes in bone mineral are more readily apparent in cancellous areas. Disparate loss of bone occurs in disuse osteoporosis, which is more obvious in cancellous regions of the skeleton, and in steroid therapy (or in primary Cushing's disease) where loss of bone mineral occurs mainly in the axial or central skeleton but not to any great extent in the peripheral skeleton.

LUCENCY.   This implies increased transradiancy of the skeleton as seen on a radiograph. This may be solitary or cystic (Table 1-2), multiple (Table 1-3), generalized leading to osteopenia (Table 1-4), or patchy, which, for example, is a common presentation of metastases from breast carcinoma.

SCLEROSIS (OR OSTEOBLASTIC).   This implies an increased density of the skeleton as seen radiographically that may be solitary (Table 1-5), multiple (Table 1-6), or generalized (Table 1-7). But one should keep in mind that it is possible to have a mixed lucent and sclerotic pattern which is exemplified by many types of metastases as well as by Paget's disease.

Table 1-2

Solitary Lucent Area

Bone cyst*
Nonossifying fibroma (fibrocortical defect)*
Enchondroma*
Cyst in association with gout or subchondral
   cysts in degenerative arthritis*
Fibrous dysplasia*
Brown tumor or hyperparathyroidism
Histiocytosis X
Giant cell tumor
Aneurysmal bone cyst
Solitary myeloma – plasmacytoma
Metastasis from hypernephroma, thyroid,
   lung, colon*

More common causes.

Table 1-3

Multiple Lucencies

Metastases: breast, lung*
Multiple myeloma*
Brown tumors of hyperparathyroidism
Eosinophilic granuloma
Arthritis, if adjacent to joints*

More common causes.

Table 1-4

Generalized Osteopenia

Osteoporosis*
Osteomalacia*
Steroids (and Cushing's disease)*
Multiple myeloma

More common causes.

Table 1-5

Solitary Sclerotic Lesions of Bone

Solid	Irregular	Solitary Dense (Ivory) Vertebra
Bone island*	Old enchondroma*	Hemangioma*
Osteoma	Bone infarct*	Paget's disease*
Osteoid osteoma	Paget's disease*	Metastases (prostate usually)*
Paget's disease (a rare form of this common condition)		Lymphoma (Hodgkin's disease)*
Eosinophilic granuloma		Rare infections
Sclerosing osteomyelitis of Garre		
Solitary metastasis (e.g., from prostate)*		

More common causes.

Table 1-6

Multiple Separate Areas of Sclerosis

Solid	Irregular
Multiple bone islands (osteopoikilosis)	Multiple metastases*
Osteopathia striata (congenital metaphyseal striations, which is rare)	Paget's disease*
Multiple osteomas (Gardner's syndrome, which is rare)	
Tuberous sclerosis (rare)	
Multiple infarcts	
Multiple metastases (prostate in men and breast in women)	

More common causes.

Table 1-7

Generalized Sclerosis of All Visualized Bones (Osteosclerosis)

Osteopetrosis (Marble bone disease,
  Albers–Schoenberg disease)
Englemann's disease (mainly cortical
  and rare)
Fluorosis
Heavy metal poisoning
Hypervitaminosis D in children
Renal bone disease*
Primary hyperparathyroidism
Myelosclerosis (myelofibrosis)*
Sickle cell anemia (rare presentation)
Multiple metastases (prostate and lung
  in men, breast in women)*
Multiple myeloma, lymphoma, leukemia
  (rare manifestation)

More common causes.

REFERENCES

Standard Texts

Edeiken J, Hodes PJ: Roentgen Diagnosis of Diseases of Bone. Baltimore, Williams & Wilkins, 1973
Greenfield GB: Radiology of Bone Diseases. Philadelphia, Lippincott, 1969
Murray RO, Jacobson HG: The Radiology of Skeletal Disorders. Edinburgh, Churchill Livingstone, 1977

Bone Morphology

Jowsey J: Metabolic Diseases of Bone. Philadelphia, Saunders, 1977
McLean FC, Urist MR: Bone. Chicago, University of Chicago Press, 1968
Vaughan JM: The Physiology of Bone. Oxford, Clarendon Press, 1975

Bone Cells

Rasmussen H, Bordier P: The cellular basis of metabolic bone disease. N Engl J Med 289:25–32, 1973
Rasmussen H, Bordier P, Kurokawa K, et al: Hormonal control of skeletal and mineral homeostasis. Am J Med 56:751–758, 1974
Whalen JP: The resorption of bone and its control: Its roentgen significance. Radiology 113:257–266, 1974

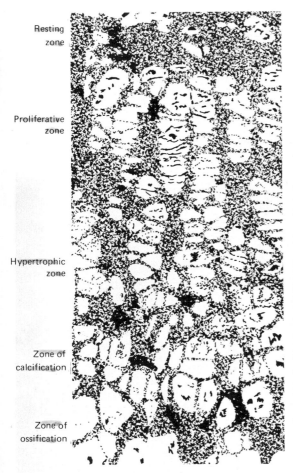

FIGURE 1-1. The zones of the physeal plate.

Resting zone

Proliferative zone

Hypertrophic zone

Zone of calcification

Zone of ossification

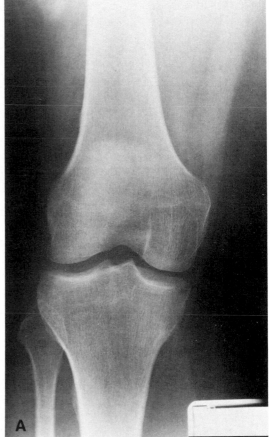

A

FIGURE 1-2. *Tubulation.* **A.** The normal configuration of the epiphysis, metaphysis, and diaphysis of the knee can be seen in this 20-year-old male with medial meniscus tear. There is no bony abnormality. (See following page for Figs. 1-2B, C.)

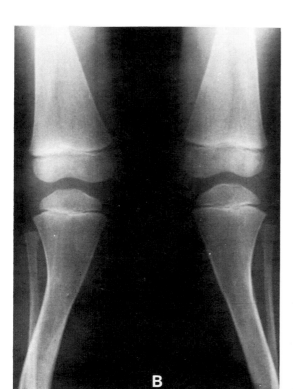

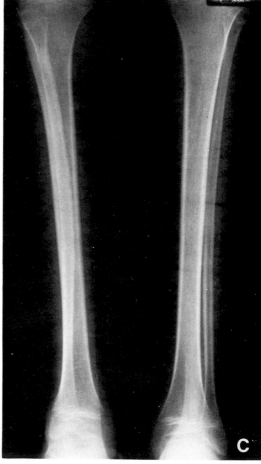

FIGURE 1-2B. Undertubulation leads to failure of remodeling of the metaphysis with this characteristic flared appearance (Erlenmeyer flask deformity). This patient has Pyle's disease which is a metaphyseal dysplasia. C. Overtubulation occurs in disuse and paralysis and the diaphysis of the bones appear narrow (gracile) as can be seen in this child with poliomyelitis. Note the almost total lack of soft tissues.

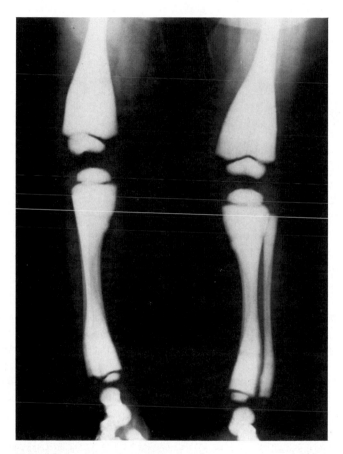

FIGURE 1-3.   Failure of endosteal osteoclasis, which is known as osteopetrosis. In these children, there is an almost total failure of both periosteal (hence the Erlenmeyer flask deformity) and endosteal osteoclasis so that no bone marrow cavity is apparent. Note the overall increase in density of the bones.

TWO

Congenital Anomalies

It is outside the scope of this book to go into great detail on many different types of congenital anomalies. Congenital and developmental defects of the limbs and long bones include reduplications, absence (phocomelia), and congenital amputations (Fig. 2-1), as well as pseudoarthroses and bones that are the wrong size, shape, or position (Fig. 2-2). Congenital anomalies of joints include congenital dislocation of the hip (see Chap. 9) and subluxations at the wrist, as well as anomalies of the spine leading to scoliosis or kyphosis including agenesis or partial failure of vertebral bodies, fused vertebrae, and hemivertebrae (Fig. 2-3).

Spina bifida is a common congenital anomaly of the spine which occurs in approximately 5 percent of the population. Although it is normally without significance, spina bifida may be associated with bulging of the meninges and is then known as a meningomyelocele, which often has serious associated abnormalities of the bladder and rectum. Scoliosis (or lateral bending of the spine) may be congenital or acquired (idiopathic or structural), and will not be dealt with further in this book. Spondylolysis and spondylolisthesis are considered in the next chapter. Kyphosis (forward bending usually of the thoracic spine) may be congenital or acquired and is considered briefly under Scheuermann's disease in Chapter 9.

Congenital anomalies in the foot can lead to many abnormalities including clubfoot, vertical talus, and metatarsus varus. The angle between the talus and the os calcis in both the anteroposterior (AP) and lateral views should be about 35° (Fig. 2-4). On the lateral view, if a line is drawn through the body of the talus it should transect the line of the metatarsals. A flat calcaneum, (i.e., the talar and calcaneal lines become parallel) leads to flat feet and a highly angled calcaneus (i.e., the talocalcaneal angle may be increased up to over 60°) leads to a clubfoot. If the talus becomes vertical (i.e., the talocalcaneal angle is 60° again but for a different reason), other specific problems occur. On the AP view, a line through the os calcis should go through the fourth metatarsal, and a line through the talus should go through or near to the first metatarsal. Deviations from this radiographic appearance are associated with clubfoot, flat feet, and varus deformities in neonates. For a fuller description of these conditions the reader is referred to the recent book by Ozonoff (see references).

Congenital anomalies may be single or may be associated with other abnormalities of the skeleton, heart, or viscera, in which case they may fall into a specific pattern known as *dysplasia*. These generalized abnormal skeletal syndromes may be classified in several ways. The pathologist, for example, will classify them depending on the abnormal tissue involved: chondroid, osteoid, or fibrous (Table 2-1). It is probably more logical, however, to approach them from their appearance on radiographs. Thus, epiphyseal, metaphyseal, and diaphyseal dysplasias are described. Finally, if these dysplasias (which involve primarily the growing ends and physeal plates of long bones) are associated with spinal anomalies, then we use the term *spondyloepiphyseal dysplasia* for example. Because many of these dysplasias are rare, they will not be discussed any further in this book. The interested reader is referred to one of the books on dysplasias that are listed at the end of this chapter.

Two of the dysplasias and one related condition will be mentioned, however, because they act as interesting physiologic models for certain situations involving the growing skeleton:

Achondroplasia

This is an autosomal dominant condition leading to short-limbed dwarfism with characteristically normal-sized heads and bodies. The growing ends of the long bones fail to mature properly and they become short and thick with widened metaphyses (Erlenmeyer flask deformity). It is associated with some spinal anomalies including narrowed interpediculate distances in the lumbar region (leading to spinal stenosis and problems in middle age) and an abnormal sacrum.

Gaucher's Disease

This is a rare hereditary metabolic condition characterized by the accumulation of cerebrosides in the reticuloendothelial cells. Although Gaucher's disease is not technically considered to be a dysplasia, this is a

Table 2-1

The Skeletal Dysplasias

I. Dysplasias due to disturbances of chondroid production
   A. Related to abnormal maturation of growth plate chondroblasts
      1. The mucopolysaccharidoses
         a. Morquio's disease
         b. Hurler's disease
         c. Other
      2. Idiopathic
         a. Achondroplasia
         b. Metaphyseal dysostosis: Jansen type, Schmid type, Spahr type
         c. Other
   B. Related to heterotopic proliferation of epiphyseal chondroblasts
      1. Enchondromatosis (Ollier's disease)
      2. Osteochondromatosis
      3. Epiphyseal hyperplasia (Fairbank)
II. Dysplasias due to disturbances in osteoid production
   A. Related to abnormal epiphyseal ossification
      1. Diastrophic dwarfism
      2. Spondyloepiphyseal dysplasia
      3. Multiple epiphyseal dysplasia (Fairbank)
      4. Stippled epiphyses
   B. Related to abnormal metaphyseal and periosteal ossification
      1. Due to deficient osteoid production
         a. Osteogenesis imperfecta
      2. Due to excessive osteoid production or deficient osteolysis
         a. Osteopetrosis (Albers–Schönberg disease)
         b. Pyknodysostosis
         c. Metaphyseal dysplasia (Pyle's disease)
         d. Diaphyseal sclerosis (Englemann's disease)
         e. Melorheostosis
         f. Osteopathia striata (Voorhoeve)
         g. Osteopoikilosis
      3. Related to abnormal osteoid production
         a. Fibrous dysplasia
         b. Neurofibromatosis
         c. Pseudarthrosis
III. Miscellaneous dysplasias
   A. Dyschondrosteosis (Madelung)
   B. Marfan's syndrome
   C. Apert's syndrome
   D. Cleidocranial dysostosis
   E. Chondroectodermal dysplasia (Ellis–van Creveld syndrome)
   F. Asphyxiating thoracic dystrophy
   G. Other affections associated with dwarfism

reasonable place to discuss this condition. It is also associated with widening of the metaphyses (Erlenmeyer flask deformity) due to a failure in tubulation. These patients have bone infarcts and may present with avascular necrosis of an epiphysis, typically the femoral head.

Morquio's Syndrome (Mucopolysaccharidosis IV)

This disease also has a characteristic radiographic appearance with flattening of the vertebral bodies that have an irregular anterior margin, while the diaphyses of the long bones are widened with irregular physeal plates and epiphyses.

DIAPHYSEAL DYSPLASIAS

Osteopetrosis ("Marble Bone" Disease or Albers–Schoenberg Disease)

This is a rare condition in which there is an almost total failure of osteoclasis. There is failure of periosteal osteoclasis leading to a lack of tubulation and widening of the metaphyses producing a characteristic Erlenmeyer flask deformity in the lower femur. There is also failure of endosteal osteoclasis and hence no bone marrow cavity is formed. These children die of protracted anemia although extramedullary hematopoesis in the liver, spleen, abdomen, and paraspinal regions of the thorax will often prolong life until early adolescence.

Radiographically the bones are dense and solid with metaphyseal widening (Fig. 2-5). The osteosclerosis is generalized and involves every bone including the skull, spine, and long bones. In spite of their radiographic appearance, the bones are brittle and many stress fractures occur. There is a curious appearance to some of the major growing centers with metaphyseal stripes known as *celery stalking*. This is due to some attempted normal enchondral bone growth but with a subsequent failure of calcification and ossification.

Engelmann's Disease

This rare condition is due to a specific failure of periosteal osteoclasis so that the diaphyses of the bones become very thick, irregular, and sclerotic (Fig. 2-6). The patients have normal endosteal osteoclasis hence normal marrow cavities and are thus not anemic. The major complication of Engelmann's disease is that some bones are inclined to overgrow (such as the fibula and radius) and so surgical amputation of the end of that bone may become necessary.

Patchy Failure of Resorption

This may occur in three patterns: (1) multiple small areas of bone fail to undergo active resorption and hence resemble multiple bone islands. This condition is called *osteopoikilosis* and the bone islands are characteristically grouped around the shoulder and hip girdles although the peripheral bones are involved frequently. It has no significance although the differential diagnosis from metastases of the prostate for example may be difficult radiographically, but osteopoikilosis is negative on bone scan and there are no associated biochemical abnormalities. (2) *Osteopathia striata* or striped bone is also of no significance and is seen in the region of the major growing physeal plates such as the knee. It is due to a partial failure of osteoclasis which occurs in a linear fashion and osteopathia striata disappears with age. (3) In *melorheostosis,* it appears that liquid bone has been poured down the sides of the long bones usually in a characteristic pattern which corresponds to the dermatomes. Melorheostosis has no significance.

Although not classically considered a "dysplasia," the next condition to be discussed, osteogenesis imperfecta, is a congenital generalized bone disorder which leads to multiple fractures and deformities of long bones.

OSTEOGENESIS IMPERFECTA

Osteogenesis imperfecta is unique in that the primary abnormality is in the collagen matrix of the bone. The exact etiology is unknown but appears to be related to the metabolism of one of the trace metals, either due to dietary deficiency or because of some enzymic abnormality. The trace metals that have been held responsible for osteogenesis imperfecta include copper, tin, and zinc. Extensive studies are underway to ascertain the exact cause of this condition.

There are various ways to classify osteogenesis imperfecta, but there appears to be three distinct forms of the disorder: a congenital variety, a juvenile type, and a delayed form.

Osteogenesis Imperfecta Congenita

The infant is either stillborn or very sickly with grossly deformed limbs due to multiple fractures. Blue sclerae are also obvious (due to the basic defect in the collagen). Radiographically, there are numerous fractures of long bones (Fig. 2-7), a poorly ossified skull with multiple wormian bones and flattened vertebrae.

Juvenile Osteogenesis Imperfecta

There is an increasing incidence of fractures with a peak just before adolescence. These children also have blue sclerae and are sometimes deaf. Radiographically, there is marked osteopenia with thin cortices which are noted to be "striated" due to widened Haversian canals. There will be many fractures, old and new, some associated with excess callus formation (Fig. 2-8). The skull may show typical changes of osteogenesis imperfecta congenita.

Osteogenesis Imperfecta Tarda

This is a rare form of "matrix" disease in which the patient has few fractures as a child and then seems to become prone to fractures following very minor trauma in the 30's and 40's.

There are a number of other congenital or hereditary conditions that are considered elsewhere in this book. Hemophilia, thalassemia, and sickle cell anemia, for example, are discussed in Chapter 9. This chapter will close with the discussion of an unusual yet not uncommon condition: fibrous dysplasia.

FIBROUS DYSPLASIA

This is another condition that is presumably congenital in origin and is related to abnormal bones. It may be monostotic with only small areas of abnormality or the whole bone may be involved, or polyostotic in which case a whole limb or side of the body may be involved. If associated with sexual precocity, fibrous dysplasia is known as Albright's syndrome.

The radiographic appearances are characteristic with loss of the normal trabecular pattern, widening of the bone with scalloping of the inner surface of the cortex, and an overall smooth "ground glass" texture to the bone (Fig. 2-9A). If fibrous dysplasia occurs in a long bone there may be bowing; in a rib, fibrous dysplasia produces a "soap bubble" appearance; and if it occurs in the femoral neck, fibrous dysplasia leads to a characteristic "shepherds crook" deformity (Fig. 2-9B). The complications of fibrous dysplasia include pathologic and incremental fractures, curious irregular speckled new bone formation within the abnormal bone, and possibly an increased incidence of sarcomatous change particularly following previous radiotherapy which was a mode of treatment 30 years ago. The more localized forms of fibrous dysplasia may fill in spontaneously without any sequelae.

REFERENCES

General

Ozonoff M: Pediatric Orthopedic Radiology. Saunders Monographs in Clinical Radiology 15. Philadelphia, Saunders, 1979

Dysplasias

Felson B (ed): Dwarfs and Other Little People. Seminars of Roentgenology. New York, Grune & Stratton, 1973

Spranger JW, Langer LO, Wiedemann H-R (eds): Bone Dysplasias. Philadelphia, Saunders, 1974

Osteogenesis Imperfecta

Dickson IR, Millar EA, Veis A: Evidence for abnormality of bone-matrix proteins in osteogenesis imperfecta. Lancet 2:586–587, 1975

Falvo KA, Bullough PG: Osteogenesis imperfecta: A histometric analysis. J Bone Joint Surg 55A:275–286, 1973

Fibrous Dysplasia

Jackson WPU, Albright F, Drewry G: Metaphyseal dysplasia, epiphyseal dysplasia, diaphyseal dysplasia, and related conditions. I. Familial metaphyseal dysplasia and craniometaphyseal dysplasia; their relation to leontiasis ossea and osteopetrosis; disorders of "bone remodeling." AMA Arch Intern Med 94:871–885, 1954

Jackson WPU, Hanelin J, Albright F: Metaphyseal dysplasia, epiphyseal dysplasia, diaphyseal dysplasia, and related conditions. II. Multiple epiphyseal dysplasia; its relation to other disorders of epiphyseal development. AMA Arch Intern Med 94:886–901, 1954

Jackson WPU, Hanelin J, Albright F: Metaphyseal dysplasia, epiphyseal dysplasia, diaphyseal dysplasia, and related conditions. III. Progressive diaphyseal dysplasia. AMA Arch Intern Med 94:902–910, 1954

Warrick CK: Some aspects of polyostotic fibrous dysplasia possible hypothesis to account for the associated endocrinological changes. Clin Radiol 24:125–138, 1973

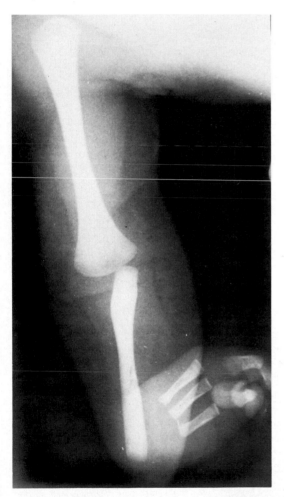

FIGURE 2-1. *Congenital absence of bone.*   This child has a radial club hand with absence of one forearm bone, two metacarpals, and three fingers. The deformity is characteristic with the solitary bone representing an "ulna" at the elbow and a "radius" at the wrist.

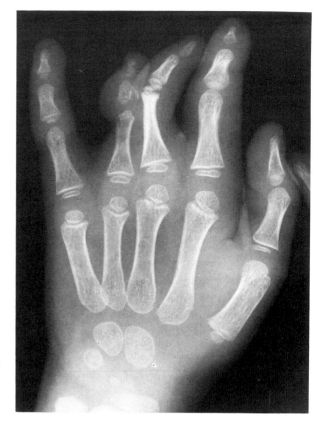

Syndactyly

FIGURE 2-2. *Congenital anomaly of the hand.* The middle and ring fingers of this child are hypoplastic, deformed, and fused. Although a rare anomaly, this is thought to be caused by amniotic fibrous bands.

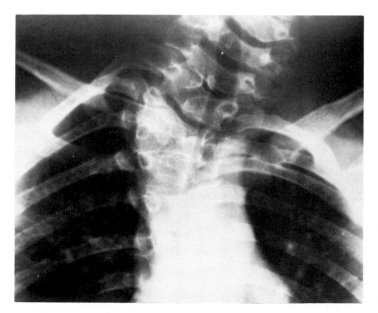

DDx Klippel-Feil

FIGURE 2-3. *Congenital scoliosis.* At the junction of the cervical and thoracic spine in this boy, a number of wedged vertebrae, hemivertebrae, and fused vertebrae may be seen leading to a curvature of the spine (scoliosis).

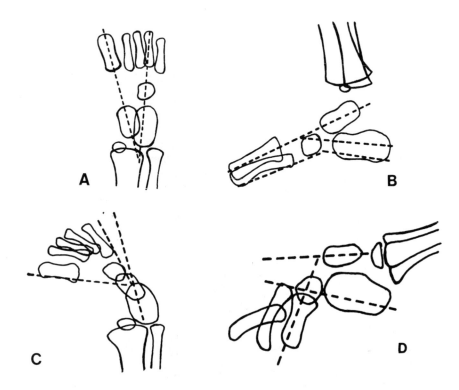

FIGURE 2-4. *Club feet.* **A, B.** Drawings of normal AP (A) and lateral views (B) of the feet. Note that the talar calcaneal angle is about 35° in both views with the line from the talus on the AP view going through the first metatarsal and that of the os calsis on the AP view going through the fourth metatarsal. On the lateral view, the talar line should go through the metatarsals. **C, D.** Club foot. In the AP view (C), the talar calcaneal angle is reversed and the midtalar line goes outside the fifth metatarsal. On the lateral view (D), the talar calcaneal angle is less than 10° with the metatarsals lying almost vertically in comparison to the talar line.

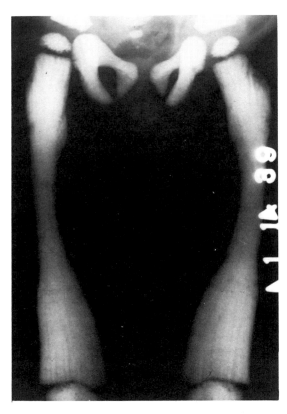

FIGURE 2-5. *Osteopetrosis.* Note the Erlenmeyer flask deformities, celery stalking, and extreme density of all the visualized bones in this child who was severely anemic due to failure of formation of the marrow cavity.

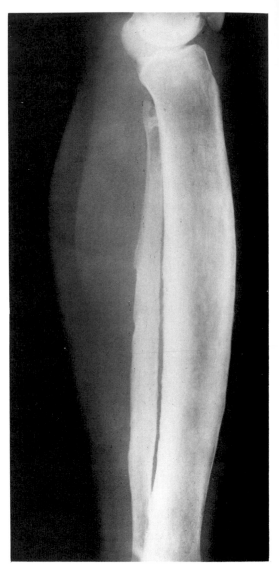

FIGURE 2-6. *Engelmann's disease.* In this condition, endosteal osteoclasis is normal, but periosteal osteoclasis has failed. Thus, the bone marrow cavities are present but there is irregular periosteal new bone growth of the long bones. Note that surgical amputation of the heads of the fibulae was necessary due to excessive overgrowth.

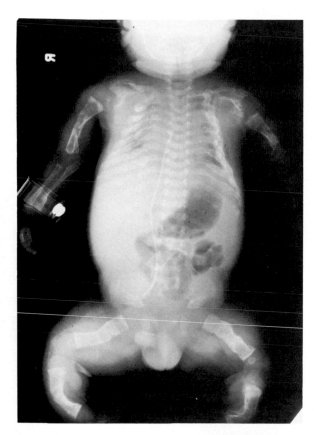

FIGURE 2-7. *Osteogenesis imperfecta congenita.* This child was stillborn; note the poor expansion of the lungs. There are multiple fractures and deformities of most of the bones in the body.

FIGURE 2-8. *Juvenile osteogenesis imperfecta.* There is poor mineralization of all the bones, and there is evidence of an old fracture of the left femur. The right femur has also been fractured and there is exuberant dense callus formation around the fracture site.

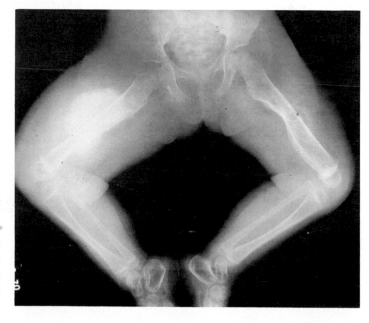

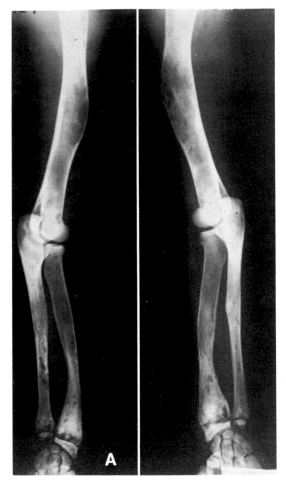

FIGURE 2-9. *Fibrous dysplasia.* **A.** Generalized form. In this young patient, many areas of localized expansion and loss of bone can be seen often with a "ground glass" appearance particularly in the radii. Note that there is sparing of parts of the long bones and some areas are actually increased in density. This is a characteristic appearance of fibrous dysplasia.

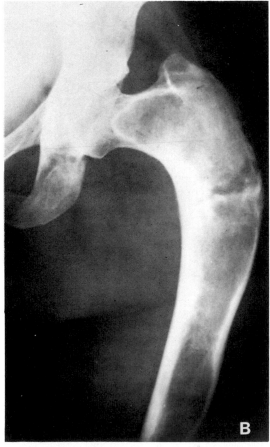

Figure 2-9B. Shepherd's crook deformity. Note the bowing and widening of the upper femur with a characteristic curve to the femoral neck and trochanteric region (shepherd's crook). An incremental fracture has occurred on the outer aspect of the upper femur.

THREE

Trauma

It is obviously unrealistic to cover every type of fracture and dislocation in a short introductory chapter on trauma, but it is important to remember some basic principles with respect to the radiographic description and appearance of fractures. The principles will be discussed initially and then some of the more common fractures will be mentioned to illustrate our basic concepts and approach to trauma.

Clinically, skeletal trauma is always associated with *soft tissue injury,* and, in some cases, this might be life-threatening (such as in fractures of the sacrum where an iliac artery may be torn) or in patients with fractures of the femoral shaft (who may lose 3 or 4 pints of blood rapidly). Nerves and vessels may be caught in between bony fragments and prolonged dislocation may lead to nerve damage or paralysis at the shoulder and hip. Fractures and dislocations may be associated with the late occurrence of avascular necrosis, the risk of which increases the longer the joint is dislocated. It is important to consider the badly traumatized patient as a whole rather than as a separate medical or orthopedic problem. For instance, fractured ribs are associated frequently with pneumothoraces or a contused lung; and fractures of the lower ribs are often associated with rupture of a viscus in the abdomen, especially the spleen, liver, or kidney. Fractures of the spine and their complications will be dealt with separately later in this chapter.

Radiologically some important theoretical and practical points should be remembered:

1. Always get *more than one view* of a traumatized area and particularly with respect to trauma of the shoulder and hip. In the

shoulder, a transaxillary view or an oblique view of the scapula will often demonstrate posterior dislocations of the shoulder, which are otherwise unsuspected (Fig. 3-1).

2. If one of *two parallel bones* is involved, or if a "ring of bone" is fractured in one place such as the pelvis, always look for a second fracture. This refers to the radius and ulna, tibia and fibula, pelvis, orbit, maxillary antrum, and even possibly to the skull itself. Particularly check the proximal fibula if there is a fracture of the distal tibia (Fig. 3-2).

3. Examine the patient carefully because in the face of major trauma to one area, it is easy to miss *other fractures*. If necessary resort to fluoroscopy or a multiple spot film technique to radiograph the whole body as is done in some Swiss and Scandinavian trauma centers.

4. Always x-ray the *full length* of a long bone from the proximal joint to the distal articulation, i.e., the hip joint down to the knee for the full length of the femur.

5. Look at the radiographs for the alignment and displacement of the bones and for associated fractures and dislocations. If you are having problems interpreting what you see, remember that techniques other than plain film radiography are usually available, such as fluoroscopy for imaging, tomography to confirm or exclude a fracture (particularly of the cervical spine), CT scanning to show the alignment of complex fractures (particularly around the shoulder girdle, hip joint, pelvis, and possibly the spine). Angiography is useful to show any bleeding points or ruptured vessels, but it is also extremely helpful in occluding a bleeding vessel by selectively introducing blood clot or gel foam in an attempt to obstruct that vessel.

The basic concept of the treatment of fractures is to reduce the fracture or dislocation and return the alignment to as near normal as possible. This is not always possible, however, bones will remodel readily in young people and if exact alignment cannot be achieved, then attempt to get two periosteal surfaces close together so that the bone can remodel and in due course it may be almost impossible to spot the previous fracture site (Fig. 3-3). Unfortunately, less remodeling occurs in adults, so it is more important then to achieve the best alignment possible during the initial few days following the injury.

Some Common Pediatric Fractures

GREENSTICK FRACTURES.   Children under the age of 12 do not always get a transverse fracture of a long bone. One cortex fractures but the other appears to bend (Fig. 3-4). Histologically, in fact, there is a fracture of the other cortex which may either be invisible or impacted. Greenstick fractures occur because the periosteum in a child is considerably thicker and stronger than that in an adult and one side bends rather than breaks. These are called greenstick fractures because the break is similar to that seen in a "green stick."

TORUS FRACTURES.   These are impaction fractures that also occur in young children (Fig. 3-5). The word *torus* has several meanings and derivations: engineers call a doughnut-shaped object (a ring within a ring) a "torus"; the ring around the base of a Greek column is also known as a "torus"; and botanically the word is used to describe the circular receptacle of a flower. Torus fractures occur classically in the distal radius following a fall on an outstretched hand or in the distal femur in young children who jump from heights such as trees.

SALTER FRACTURES.   In 1963, Salter divided epiphyseal fractures into five types and although his original description has been somewhat modified, it is still a useful classification (Fig. 3-6). Physeal plate fractures are important because trauma and bleeding into the growth plate may cause damage if not actual fusion and hence cessation of growth in that part of the plate. If it is localized, cone-shaped epiphyses will result (Fig. 3-7), but if the fusion is of a whole growth plate, it becomes important to take into account the age of the child and the importance of that particular growth center, i.e. the upper humerus and distal radius are responsible for the majority of the growth in the arm, but a somewhat shorter arm is of lesser importance than a short leg. Salter fractures of the distal femoral epiphysis or of either the proximal or distal tibial epiphyses (Fig. 3-8) may lead to significant shortening of that limb. If this is anticipated, it may become necessary to perform an epiphysiodesis (a physeal plate fusion) on the equivalent physeal plate of the *contralateral limb* so that the child is not left with a permanent limp.

SUPRACONDYLAR FRACTURES.   A common injury in children are fractures of the supracondylar region of the humerus. There are two points of interest about this fracture: the capsule of the elbow joint is inserted into the hollows of the distal humerus and each of these hollows contains a fat pad which acts as a buffer between the humerus and the olecranon and coronoid processes. If an effusion occurs, these fat pads, which are normally not visible, appear (Fig. 3-9A). If the fat pads become visible on the lateral view in children following trauma to the elbow, a supracondylar fracture should be suspected. In adults, a fracture of the radial head must be sought when the "fat pad sign" becomes positive. Most supracondylar fractures also result in an alteration in the alignment of the condyles to the humeral head and the condyles may come to lie directly under the shaft of the humerus (Fig. 3-9A). Oblique and AP views are often necessary to actually demonstrate the fracture (Fig. 3-9B). Following reduction of the fracture, the alignment of the condyles should return to normal, i.e., 25° in front of the line of the humeral shaft (Fig. 3-9C).

Some Common Adult Fractures

COLLES' FRACTURES.   With advancing age, bone mineral decreases and initially secondary trabeculae are lost, particularly in those parts of the skeleton which are predominantly cancellous bone. Thus, fractures of the femoral neck and distal radius become more common. In 1814, Abraham Colles described a fracture involving the distal radius and ulna with posterior displacement of the fracture fragments leading to a clinically apparent "dinner fork deformity" (Fig. 3-10). The alignment of the radial shaft to the radiocarpal joint is abnormal and what is normally a 15° anterior angulation often becomes a 30° posterior angulation, and this should be reduced as close to normal as possible.

FEMORAL NECK FRACTURES.   These are classified depending on the level of the fracture (Fig. 3-11) and are important because the more proximal the fracture, the greater the incidence of avascular necrosis. Often elderly and female patients are admitted after having fallen. They complain of pain in the hip and the leg will be shortened and internally rotated. Usually the diagnosis can be made on a straight AP view of the pelvis (Fig. 3-12), but it is sometimes necessary to take oblique and lateral views of the upper femur or to resort to stereoscopy or even tomography to confirm the diagnosis.

PELVIC FRACTURES.   The pelvis acts as a "ring of bone" and often "entrance" (pubic and ischael rami) and "exit" (sacrum or sacroiliac joint diastasis) fractures are present. It is very important to look for these since sacral abnormalities are easy to miss. The fractures of the rami and separation of the symphysis are often associated with severe soft tissue damage, particularly to the bladder and urethra. Fractures of the sacrum or separation of the sacroiliac joints may be associated with damage to the iliac vessels (Fig. 3-13).

Other Types of Fractures

AVULSION FRACTURES.   These fractures occur at sites of muscle origin and can be seen in both children and adults. The classic example in an adult is a fracture of the olecranon with separation of the fragments as the triceps contracts (Fig. 3-14). Another common site, particularly in baseball players, is an avulsion fracture of the ischial tuberosity (Fig. 3-15) due to tearing of the insertion of the hip adductors.

STRESS FRACTURES.   To some extent all fractures are caused by stress but the term *stress fractures* refers to an abnormal stress such as is seen in athletes; for instance, the tibia in joggers and ballet dancers; the metatarsals in people who walk or march excessively ("march fracture"); and the humeral neck in soldiers or backpackers who carry heavy loads on their shoulders. It is often impossible to see the fracture initially (Figs. 3-16A, 3-17A), but a bone scan will be positive within 48 hours of a fracture, stress or otherwise. A periosteal reaction, bone resorption, and callus can be seen from 3 to 6 weeks later depending on the bone involved (Figs. 3-16B, 3-17B).

PATHOLOGIC FRACTURES.   Any process that leads to an inherent weakening of the bone will lead to "pathologic" fractures or fractures through a pathologic abnormality. The process may be benign and occur in children (Fig. 3-18) or adults (Fig. 3-19). Patients with osteogenesis imperfecta have many fractures (see Chap. 2), and, of course, patients with osteoporosis also fracture more easily than patients without loss of bone mineral. One could consider, therefore, all fractures in patients over the age of 60 to be "pathologic" in a sense but in fact the term is reserved for more localized pathologic situations. The most common cause of pathologic fractures is undoubtedly the metastatic spread of cancer, particularly from a primary in the breast in women and in the lung in men. Not infrequently, a patient presents with a fracture of a long bone which turns out to have an unsuspected underlying pathologic process which leads to the fractures (Fig. 3-20).

Dislocations

The definition of a *dislocation* is when two normally contiguous joint surfaces are displaced and are no longer in contact. *Subluxations* are incomplete dislocations and are most often seen in association with ligamentous laxity and in rheumatoid arthritis. Dislocations usually follow trauma and may involve any joint in the body although one possible exception to this traumatic etiology is in congenital dislocation of the hip (see Chap. 9). The majority of dislocations have few sequelae once they have been reduced, particularly if the reduction is rapid and complete. Some dislocations, however, are associated with major complications. These include, for example, dislocations of the *elbow* in which nerves may become trapped or vessels may get torn, and in dislocations of the *hip* where the longer the femoral head is out of the acetabulum, the greater the risk of avascular necrosis. A number of specific dislocations will be discussed briefly.

SHOULDER.   Of all dislocations of the shoulder, 95 percent are anterior, and the humeral head slips downwards and medially making it easy to diagnose both clinically and radiologically (Fig. 3-21). The remaining 5 percent of shoulder dislocations present a problem because the head slips straight back posteriorly and on AP radiographs appears to still lie in the glenoid (Fig. 3-1), and thus an x-ray in a different plane is essential. This may be taken transthoracically as an axial view or as an oblique view.

WRIST.   There are two classic dislocations at the radiocarpal joint: the *perilunate dislocation* in which the lunate and radius remain in proximity whereas all the other carpal bones dislocate around the lunate (Fig. 3-22A,B) or the *lunate dislocation* in which the lunate dislocates anteriorly by itself (Fig. 3-22C).

ACROMIOCLAVICULAR DISLOCATIONS.   These are also common and easily diagnosed clinically and confirmed by giving the patient weights to hold and hence pulling down on the acromion and demonstrating the dislocation.

Complications, of Trauma, Fractures, and Dislocations

LIGAMENTOUS DAMAGE.   Ligamentous damage varies from complete tears such as occur in the ankle or with subtalar dislocations, to ligamentous laxity leading to recurrent dislocations, for example, in the shoulder where a notch occurs on the upper surface of the proximal part of the greater tuberosity (a "Hill Sachs" deformity) due to recurrent impingment of the humeral head on the lower surface of the glenoid labrum (Fig. 3-21). Occasionally a damaged ligament will calcify as a result of internal hemorrhage and the classic example of this is at the knee—the so-called Pelligrini Stieda calcification (Fig. 3-23).

DAMAGE TO THE ARTICULAR CARTILAGE LEADING TO PREMATURE ARTH-RITIS.   This is particularly true of the weight-bearing joints, and, for instance, fractures of the upper tibia are very often associated with separation of the tibial plateaus and an altered relationship between the weight-bearing surfaces of the femoral condyles and the tibia leading to early degenerative arthritis (Fig. 3-24).

MYOSITIS OSSIFICANS.   This may occur in muscles that become traumatized; it was in fact first described in the 18th century in fractures of the elbow in young women who fell off their horses while hunting. Myositis ossificans is particularly common at points of muscle insertion and origin in the upper leg. The diagnosis is often difficult to substantiate initially although a bone scan is often positive within 48 hours, but at least 3 weeks pass before there are any radiographic changes. There is slow maturation of the ossification, taking from 6 to 18 months (Fig. 3-25A). Two types of ectopic bone formation are important because their appearance is confusing: (1) In trauma to the periosteum, bleeding and periosteal reaction may occur which may be difficult to differentiate from an osteosarcoma (Fig. 3-25B) and represents a periosteal hemorrhage. (2) At the insertion of the vastus mediallus, it is not uncommon to see an irregular periosteal reaction (Fig. 3-25C), and it closely resembles an osteogenic sarcoma on biopsy. So before the leg is amputated, x-ray the other side for comparison and if that is normal, wait 3 to 4 weeks and then x-ray the involved side again: a *metaphyseal cortical defect* will be unchanged whereas a true osteogenic sarcoma will have enlarged.

AVASCULAR NECROSIS. Although there are many causes of avascular necrosis (Tables 3-1, 3-2), the most common is trauma either following a fracture of the femoral neck or a dislocation of the femoral or humeral head. The radiographic appearances of avascular necrosis can vary but the earliest sign is often a "crescent" sign (Fig. 3-26A), which represents a subchondral fracture through the insertion of the individual trabeculae, which are infarcted, and the subchondral bone, which receives much of its nutrients from the synovial fluid and overlying cartilage. Ultimately, this also collapses and with further collapse of the infarcted bone marked distortion occurs (Fig. 3-26B). Areas of dead bone can appear normal radiographically and do not change density except either when the bone impacts or when reactive new bone is laid down alongside the dead trabeculae.

The carpal navicular bone (scaphoid) receives its blood supply predominantly from its distal pole so that fractures of the waist of the navicular can result in avascular necrosis of the proximal pole. This occurs in about 30 percent of fractures of the navicular and is seen radiographically as increasing sclerosis of the proximal pole (Fig. 3-27). Avascular necrosis may stabilize itself and even heal to a large extent if weight bearing is curtailed or if the area is immobilized.

Trauma Involving the Spine

Severe damage to the vertebral column is often associated with damage to the spinal cord and hence spinal cord injury and paralysis (either quadriplegia or paraplegia depending on the level of the injury) will occur. Thus, it is very important to exercise extreme caution in the management

Table 3-1

The Etiology of Osteonecrosis

Posttraumatic
  1. Fractures
  2. Dislocations
  3. Microfractures
Nontraumatic
  A. Embolic
    1. Hemoglobinopathies, sickle cell disease, sickle cell trait, and sickle cell thalassemia
    2. Decompression states and caisson disease
    3. Pancreatitis
    4. Alcoholism
  B. Small Vessel Disease
    1. Connective tissue disorders: polyarteritis, systemic lupus erythematosus, giant cell arteritis, Fabry's disease
  C. Abnormal Deposition of Cells
    1. Gaucher's disease
    2. Steroid therapy
    3. Cushing's disease
Other Conditions—"Idiopathic"
  1. In association with degenerative arthritis
  2. Gout and hyperuricemia
  3. Prolonged immobilization
  4. Cytotoxic therapy
  5. In association with hyperparathyroidism
  6. In association with metastases
  7. In association with lymphoma
  8. Pregnancy
  9. Multiple injuries or burns

Table 3-2

Suggested Pathogenesis of Osteonecrosis

Emboli and Infarcts
  1. Fat
  2. Nitrogen
  3. Vascular
Mechanical
  1. Fractures and dislocations
  2. Osteoarthritis
Infiltration with abnormal cells
  1. Gaucher's
  2. Steroids and Cushing's disease
Bleeding Disorders
  1. Hypercoagulability: eg. alcoholism
  2. Hypocoagulability
Fat Necrosis
  1. Pancreatitis

of patients with suspected spinal injury. An AP and cross table lateral radiograph of the part of the spine involved should be taken without moving the patient. The alignment of the vertebral bodies, the spinal canal, facet joints, and posterior elements must be studied (Fig. 3-28), and if there is any malalignment, some form of brace or a halo must be applied before the patient can be moved. This is particularly important in the cervical region where fracture dislocations or whiplash injuries are not uncommon following motor vehicle accidents. If there is any doubt with regard to whether there is a fracture present or not, tomography is helpful. Flexion and extension views can be useful as long as they are done with extreme care and the patient's clinical state is monitored continuously. More recently, the CT scanner has also proven to be a useful tool in assessing fractures particularly of the lumbar spine.

This is an appropriate place to mention *spondylolysis* and *spondylolisthesis*. *Spondylolysis* means a break (lysis) in the spinal arch and in fact refers to a defect in the pars interarticularis of one or more of the lower lumbar vertebral arches posteriorly. It can be best seen on an oblique view where the "scotty dog" appears to have a collar across his neck (Fig. 3-29). Spondylolysis is found in about 5 percent of the population with or without backache. It appears to be caused by a series of stress fractures probably due to long-standing rotatory stress on this part of the spinal ring in young children with a genetic tendency to have a narrower pars than normal.

Spondylolisthesis, on the other hand, refers to the anterior slippage of one vertebral body on the one below and is often associated with symptoms. In order for a slip to occur either bilateral spondylolysis or ligamentous laxity must be present. The incidence of spondylolithesis is similar to spondylolysis (about 5 percent of the population) and usually occurs in the lower lumbar region or at the lumbosacral junction. It is often classified by the degree of the slip into grades I, II, and III, each one referring to one-third of the depth of the vertebral bodies involved (Fig. 3-30). Degenerative spondylolisthesis is seen in elderly patients with progressive degenerative disc disease and is always associated with disc space narrowing. *Retrolisthesis* is a reversed spondylolisthesis and is usually associated with trauma or degenerative disc disease.

REFERENCES

Bowerman JW: Radiology and Injury in Sport. New York, Appleton, 1977

Salter RB, Harris WR: Injuries involving the epiphyseal plate. J Bone Joint Surg 45-A:587–621, 1963

Watson-Jones R: Fractures and joint injuries. Edinburgh, Churchill Livingstone, 1976

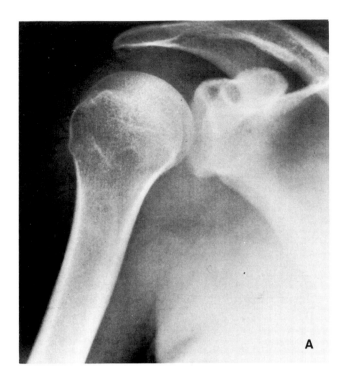

FIGURE 3-1. *Posterior dislocation of the shoulder.* **A.** AP view. **B.** Transaxillary view. Although the AP view initially appears unremarkable, in fact, there is too much separation between the glenoid fossa and the humeral head. The transaxillary view confirms the posterior dislocation (C = *coracoid,* G = *glenoid,* H = *humeral head).*

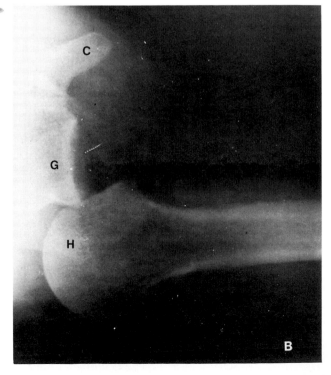

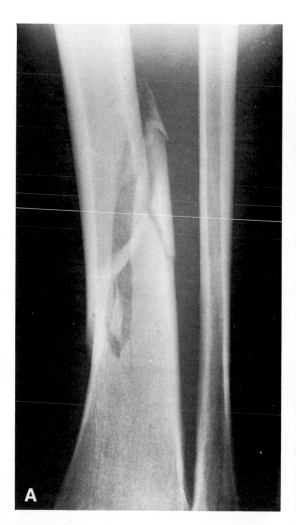 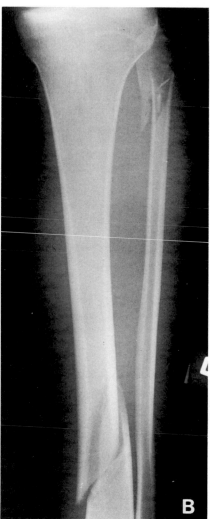

FIGURE 3-2. *Unsuspected fracture of proximal fibula.* **A.** AP ankle. **B.** AP lower leg. This 24-year-old male fell of his motorcycle at high speed and initial views of the ankle demonstrated a comminuted spiral fracture of the distal tibia. A full length radiograph revealed the associated fracture of the proximal fibula.

FIGURE 3-3. *Healing, repair, and remodeling in a 10-year-old boy.*   **A.** The initial film shows rather poor alignment of the fracture fragments in this oblique fracture of the distal femur. **B.** Seven weeks later there is obvious callus formation and buttressing from one periosteal surface to the other. Note the rounding off of the edges of the fracture fragments. (See facing page for Figs. 3-3C, D.)

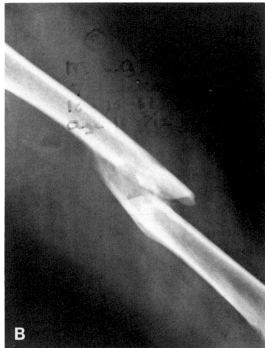

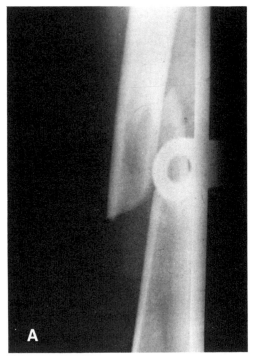

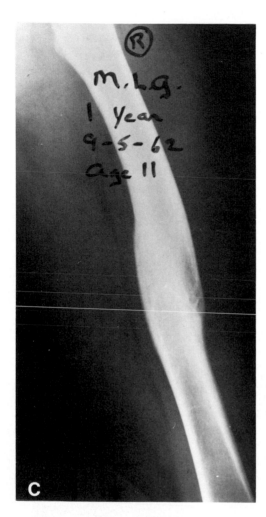

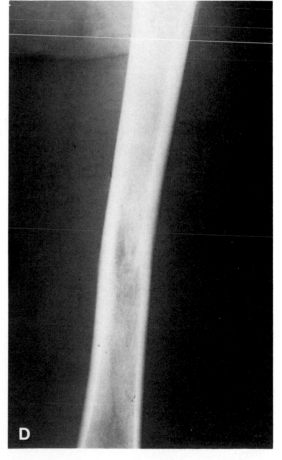

Figure 3-3C. At 1 year, there has been considerable remodeling and healing with nearly complete restoration of alignment. **D.** At 2 years, the fracture site is almost invisible although there is a slight bend in the femur with a central lucency at the original site.

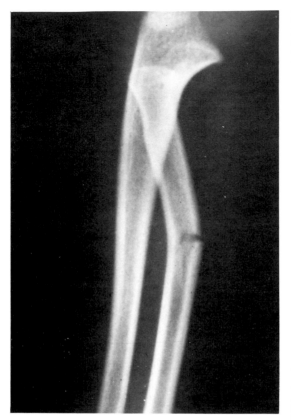

FIGURE 3-4. *Greenstick fracture.* There is a typical greenstick fracture of the radius in this young child with a fracture through one cortex and apparent bending of the other.

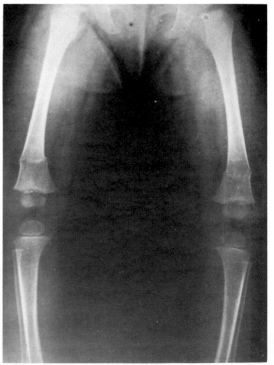

FIGURE 3-5. *Torus fracture.* This child fell from a tree and has sustained symmetrical impaction buckling fractures of both lower femurs (torus fractures).

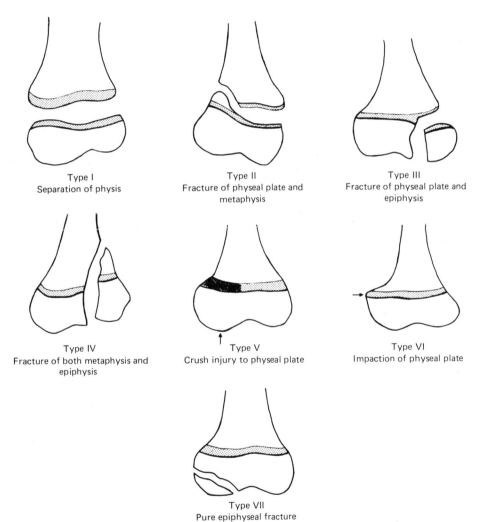

Type I
Separation of physis

Type II
Fracture of physeal plate and
metaphysis

Type III
Fracture of physeal plate and
epiphysis

Type IV
Fracture of both metaphysis and
epiphysis

Type V
Crush injury to physeal plate

Type VI
Impaction of physeal plate

Type VII
Pure epiphyseal fracture

FIGURE 3-6. Classification of physeal plate fractures after Salter.

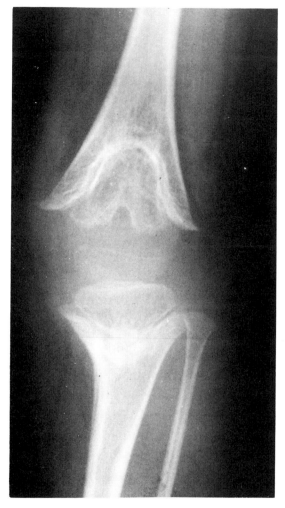

FIGURE 3-7. *Cone-shaped epiphysis.* Although many causes of cone-shaped epiphyses have been postulated, the most likely cause is probably trauma to the central portion of the physeal plate with subsequent fusion of the center and finally overgrowth of the edges leading to the characteristic "tulip" appearance.

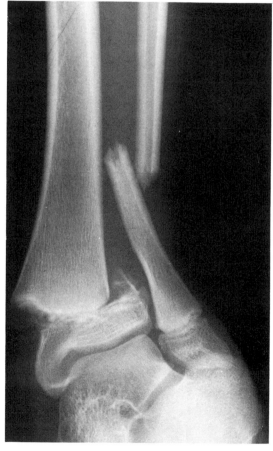

FIGURE 3-8. *Salter II fracture of the distal tibia.* Note the disruption of the physeal plate with the small separated fragment of the tibial metaphysis laterally. The fibula is fractured above the physeal plate in this 12-year-old boy who fell off his bike.

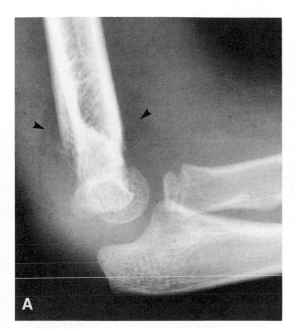

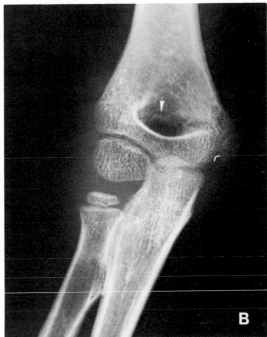

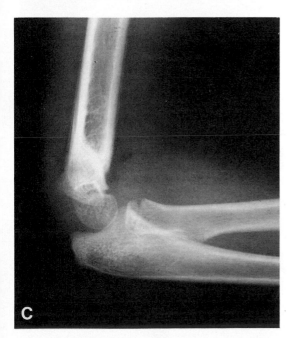

FIGURE 3-9. *Supracondylar fracture of the elbow.* **A.** Initial lateral view showing displacement of the fat pads (arrows) and alteration of the alignment of the condyles and epicondyles. **B.** An oblique view shows the fracture line (arrow). **C.** Following reduction, the alignment is normal with the condyles lying some 25° in front of the humeral shaft. Note the periosteal reaction in this film taken 3 weeks after injury.

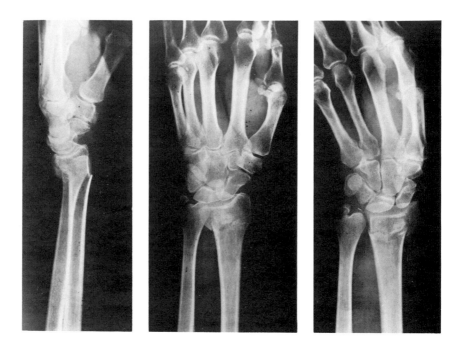

FIGURE 3-10. *Colles' fracture.*   There are fractures of the distal radius and ulna styloid with posterior displacement and a 20° posterior angulation of the distal radius on the radial shaft. Shortening of the distal radius is also noted.

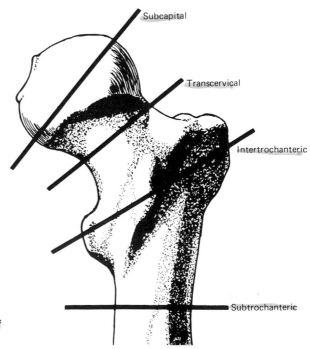

FIGURE 3-11.   A simple classification of femoral neck fractures.

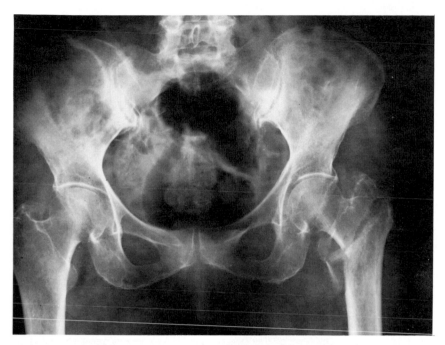

FIGURE 3-12. *Intertrochanteric fracture of the left femur in an elderly female patient with known osteoporosis.* Note the fracture line and the separation of the lesser trochanter to which the iliopsoas muscle is attached.

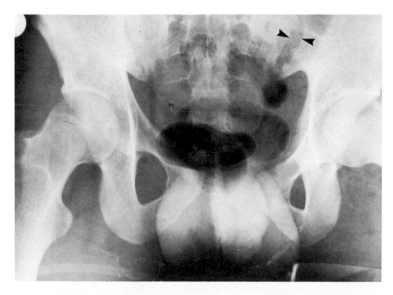

FIGURE 3-13. *Pelvic injury.* There is separation of the symphysis pubis of this 18-year-old male patient who was involved in a motor vehicle accident. He had ruptured his urethra. The other injury is to the left sacroiliac joint which is separated (arrows), although in fact he did not sustain any injury to his major vessels.

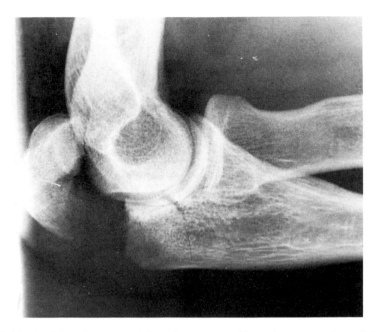

FIGURE 3-14. *Avulsion fracture of the olecranon.* Note the separation of the fracture fragments because of the pull of the triceps tendon. This is a comminuted fracture involving the joint surface.

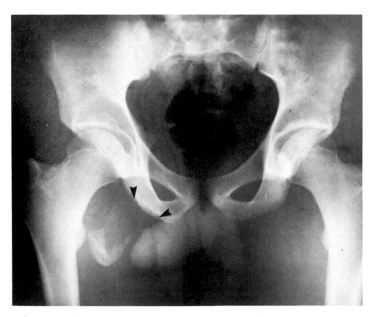

Rider's bone

FIGURE 3-15. *Avulsion fracture of the ischial tuberosity.* There is marked separation of the tuberosity from its normal site of attachment (arrows) due to muscle spasm. This has to be reduced and the tuberosity is often fixed back into place using internal fixation.

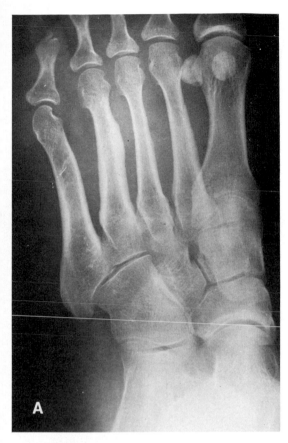

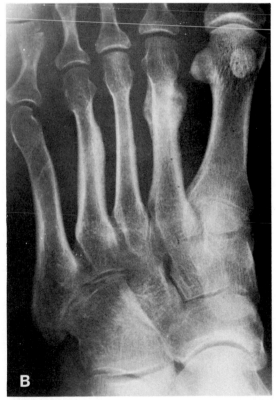

FIGURE 3-16. *Stress fracture second metatarsal.* **A.** Initial film that was passed as normal apart from evidence of an old stress fracture of the fourth metatarsal. **B.** A film taken 3 weeks later shows exuberant callus formation around the distal end of the second metatarsal. In retrospect, an oblique line can be seen running through the medial cortex at this point on the initial film.

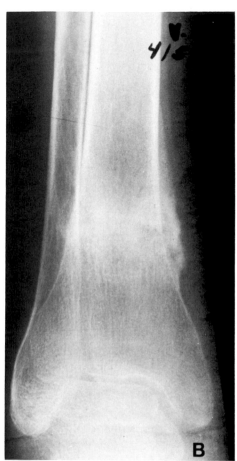

FIGURE 3-17. *Stress fracture tibia.*   **A.** The initial film on this 55-year-old ballet teacher with pain in the lower leg was read as normal. **B.** Two months later the patient presented with continuing pain and the radiograph shows both endosteal and periosteal callus formation around a stress fracture of the tibia.

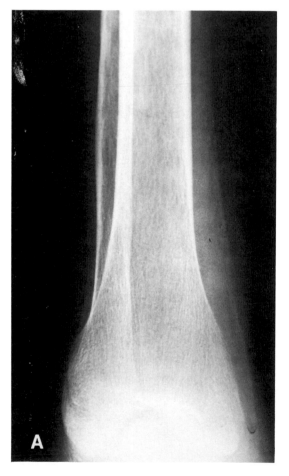

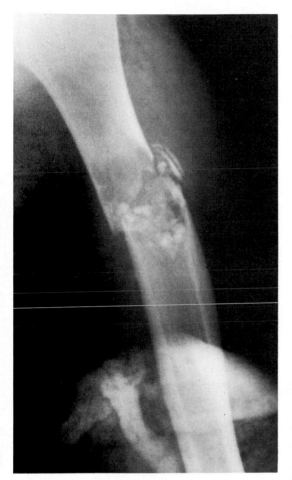

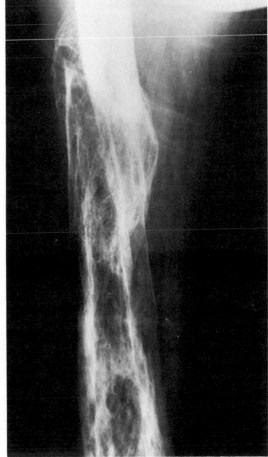

FIGURE 3-18. *Pathologic fracture through an enchondroma.* There is a comminuted transverse fracture through a benign enchondroma in this 28-year-old man. The enchondroma is typical, being lucent and containing many flocculent calcifications.

FIGURE 3-19. *Pathologic fracture in Paget's disease with healing.* This 72-year-old man felt a crack and his leg collapsed under him. A pathologic fracture through the osteolytic area of unsuspected Paget's disease had occurred. This radiograph was taken a year after the episode and demonstrates excellent callus formation, healing, and alignment.

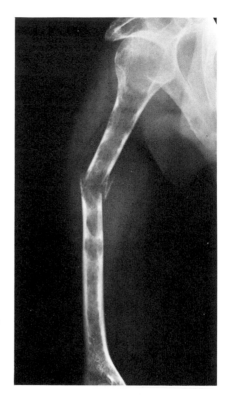

FIGURE 3-20. *Pathologic fracture through a metastatic focus in the humerus.* This 54-year-old female patient had had breast carcinoma for 3 years and had only recently developed bone metastases. The pathologic fracture occurred while positioning her on the x-ray table to take this radiograph.

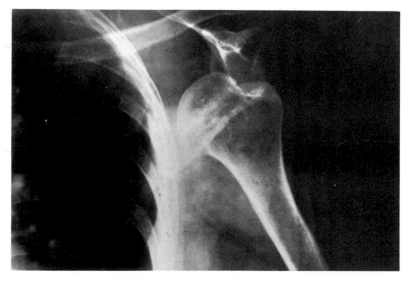

FIGURE 3-21. *Anterior dislocation of the shoulder.* The humeral head lies under the glenoid which has caused an indentation between the greater tuberosity and the head itself (a "Hill-Sachs deformity"). This is usually a sign of recurrent anterior dislocation, as it was in this patient.

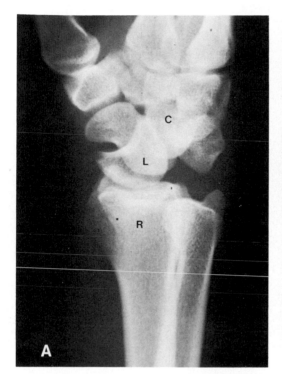

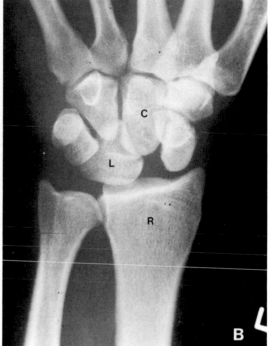

Pie wedge
sign

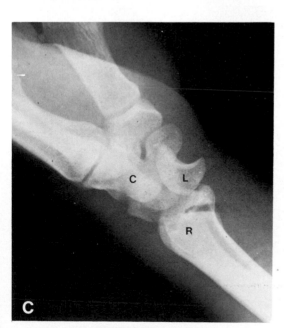

FIGURE 3-22. *Dislocation about the lunate.*   **A.** Perilunate dislocation: in this situation, the lunate (L) and the radius (R) remain in normal anatomic position and the other carpal bones dislocate posteriorly around the lunate. Note the position of the capitate (C). **B.** AP view of the same patient shows the characteristic pyramidal shape of the dislocated lunate (L). **C.** Lunate dislocation. Note that the lunate (L) lies anterior to the line of the radius (R) and capitate (C).

Orange peel sign

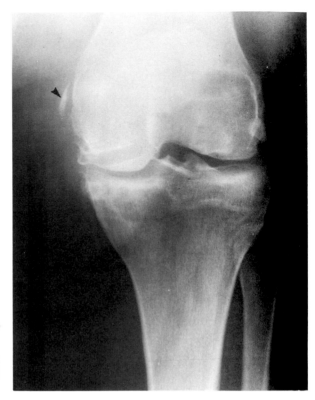

FIGURE 3-23. *"Pelligrini–Stieda" calcification in the medial collateral ligament of the knee.* Calcification in the medial collateral ligament (arrow) occurs as a result of a tear and hemorrhage into the ruptured ligament.

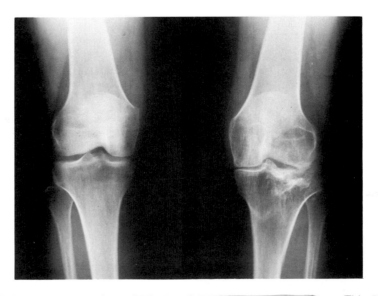

FIGURE 3-24. *Damage to the articular cartilage following a fracture.* This 54-year-old female patient had sustained a tibial plateau fracture 10 years previously. She is now complaining of pain and swelling in her left knee. The radiograph demonstrates early degenerative arthritis with joint space narrowing, sclerosis, and deformity of the tibial plateau as a result of the old fracture.

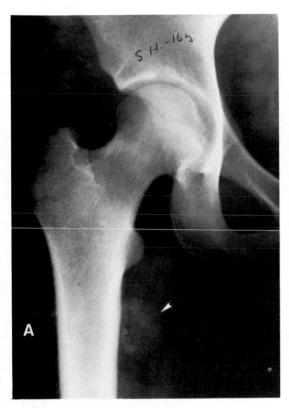

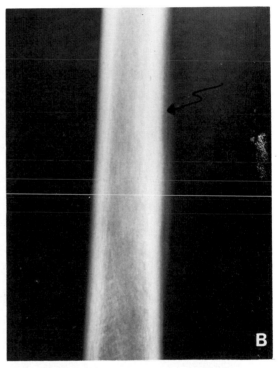

FIGURE 3-25. *Myositis ossificans.* There are a number of types of heterotopic bone formation following trauma. **A.** Classical myositis ossificans which follows trauma and bleeding into a muscle, often at its insertion, leading to subsequent ossification (arrow). **B.** Myositis ossificans resembling a parosteal osteosarcoma. This 24-year-old man complaining of pain in his leg following minor trauma had initial films that showed a diffuse periosteal reaction around the distal femur. Oblique films showed the discrete lucent line between the underlying bone and the new periosteal bone (arrow). This represents the periosteum which is fibrous tissue and hence lucent. In a parosteal osteosarcoma, the periosteum is shifted away from its original position and hence this is a good way to differentiate between the two conditions. (For Fig. 3-25C see following page.)

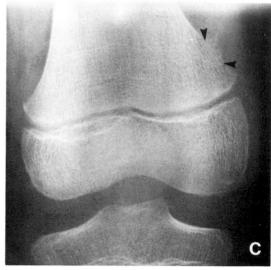

FIGURE 3-25C. *Metaphyseal cortical defect.*   Note the poorly defined myositis ossificans and the break in the cortex of the medial femoral condyle (arrows). Although this appearance is characteristic of metaphyseal cortical defects, it has to be carefully differentiated from osteosarcoma.

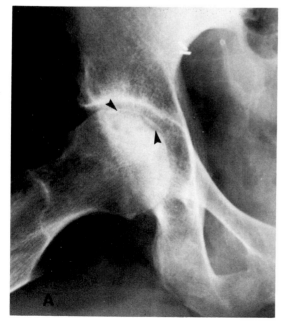

FIGURE 3-26. *Avascular necrosis of the femoral head.*   **A.** One of the earliest signs of avascular necrosis is a subchondral lucent line ("crescent" sign) best seen in a frog-leg view of the pelvis (arrows). This patient had received a renal transplant 15 months before this radiograph was taken and is on high doses of steroids. (For Fig. 3-26B see facing page.)

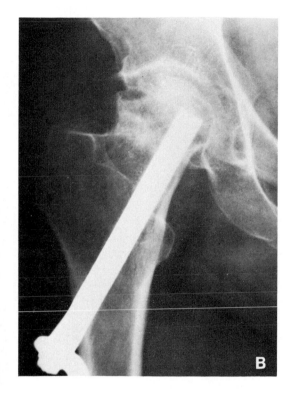

B

FIGURE 3-26B. As the condition progresses, there is collapse of the femoral head with disintegration and fragmentation leading to severe degenerative arthritis. The avascular necrosis occurred in this 58-year-old female following a transcervical fracture of the femoral neck.

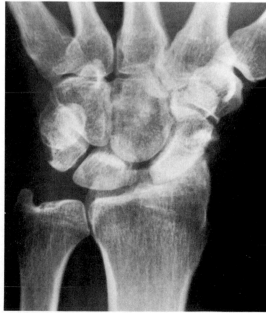

FIGURE 3-27. *Avascular necrosis secondary to a fracture of the navicular.* Note the increased density of the proximal pole of the navicular in this young woman who sustained a transverse fracture of the bone 6 months previously. This sclerosis represents avascular necrosis and is due either to impaction of dead bone or due to laying down of new bone. Note also the separation of the lunate and navicular (scapholunate disassociation) and the secondary degenerative arthritis in the radionavicular joint.

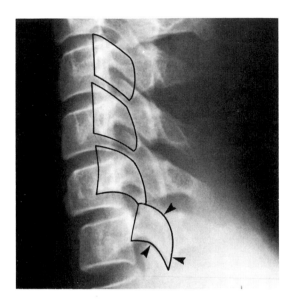

Lowtie sign

FIGURE 3-28. *Cross-table lateral view of the cervical spine.*   There is a subluxation of the lateral mass of C5 anteriorly on C6. The pillars (lateral masses) should superimpose on each other on a normal true lateral of the cervical spine (as does C6-arrows) but if there is a rotatory subluxation, they are no longer superimposed. This is a potentially fatal sitiation if not diagnosed immediately. (Marks have been placed on the subluxed pillars.)

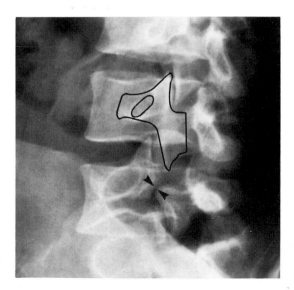

FIGURE 3-29. *Spondylolysis.*   Note the black collar (arrows) across the neck of the Scotty dog.

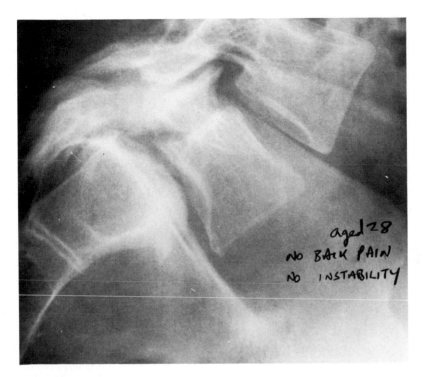

FIGURE 3-30. *Spondylolisthesis.* There is at least 1 cm anterior slippage of L5 on S1 in this 28-year-old physician who had no back pain or demonstrable instability. There is sclerosis of the superior surface of S1 with some disc space narrowing as well as relative wedging of the posterior aspect of L5 which are typical findings in spondylolisthesis.

FOUR

Infections

Infections of the musculoskeletal system may be conveniently subdivided into those involving bones (osteomyelitis) and those involving joints (septic arthritis). The spine is best considered separately.

OSTEOMYELITIS

It was thought that with the advent of antibiotics, osteomyelitis would disappear, however, this has not proven to be the case although the majority of patients who develop bone infections today are often immunosuppressed, usually either shortly after birth or from steroid therapy. But osteomyelitis also occurs in drug addicts de novo and can be seen as a late complication of diabetes (see Chap. 9). Patients with sickle cell anemia also are more prone to develop infections, presumably secondary to ischemia (possibly similar to diabetics), and this is discussed later in this chapter.

Even today, *Staphylococcus aureus* is still responsible for over 90 percent of all bone and joint infections except in immunosuppressed patients and in drug addicts who mainline. The classic site for osteomyelitis is at the junction of the epiphysis and metaphysis at the point of separation of the two separate blood supplies, that from the physeal plate and that from the more central diaphyseal nutrient artery (Fig. 4-1A). The infection begins just below the periosteum and tracks down between this and the cortex as well as running down the endosteal surface of the cortex (Fig. 4-1B). Although any long bone may be involved, classically osteomyelitis affects the humerus, femur, tibia, and fibula most commonly.

Initially, the patients present with *dolor, color, rubor,* and *tumor.* The first radiographic sign of osteomyelitis is soft-tissue swelling with loss of the fat planes (Fig. 4-2A). After about 10 days, loss of the clear-cut cortical margins occur and a periosteal reaction may be seen (Fig. 4-2B), which is rapidly followed by patchy destruction of cancellous bone and formation of periosteal new bone in an effort to wall off the infection. This new bone is known as an *involucrum* (derived from the Latin "to wrap or cover") and since the cortical bone lying within this pool of pus is avascular and dead, this is known as the *sequestrum* (derived from the Latin and a middle English legal term meaning "to seclude") (Fig. 4-2C). If the infection is still not treated, then the abscess will break down and sinus tracts occur allowing pus to drain to the surface often with holes appearing in the involucrum to allow this to happen. These holes are known as *lacunae* and this situation is then called chronic osteomyelitis (Fig. 4-3). It should be rare today although we still see veterans who have chronic osteomyelitis in a long bone such as the femur. It is very difficult to treat; even with massive long-term antibiotic therapy and with surgical intervention by scraping out the abscess cavity and removing the sequestrum, chronic osteomyelitis often recurs. It is still occasionally necessary to treat it by amputation. There are two classical complications of chronic osteomyelitis: (1) amyloidosis, (2) squamous cell metaplasia of the sinus tract leading to squamous cell carcinoma of the lining and surrounding skin.

Because the earliest positive radiographic changes are delayed at least 10 days after the start of the infection and the earlier the treatment the more rapid the response to the correct antibiotic (usually intravenous penicillin), it is necessary to diagnose an osteomyelitis as soon as possible. This is one place where bone scanning is of great help. A technetium polyphosphonate or diphosphonate scan becomes positive within the first 48 hours of the infection and is a very sensitive method for detecting early osteomyelitis. A gallium scan also becomes positive very early in an infection but is incapable of differentiating between a cellulitis and a true osteomyelitis.

Another common type of osseous infection seen today is following implantation of metal into the skeleton either as internal fixation for a fracture with pins and plates (Fig. 4-4) or following a total joint replacement where the incidence of secondary infection varies from 5 to 20 percent. This latter type of osteomyelitis can be difficult to detect, and often the bone or joint has to be aspirated before the diagnosis can be confirmed, although the patient will complain of pain and may have febrile episodes.

BRODIE'S ABSCESS

There is also a characteristic form of chronic bone abscess which is seen because either the organism is not particularly virulent or because the patient is healthy. Presumably the classic initial phases of the osteomyelitis occur although the patient is unaware of them, and the infection becomes chronic and walled off. This is known as a *Brodie's abscess* and occurs classically at the distal end of long bones such as the femur and tibia. The radiographic appearances are of a well-defined lucency with clear-cut margins in the metaphysis either actually adjacent to the physeal plate or with a small "tail" running down to the plate itself (Fig. 4-5). The patient will often have little in the way of systemic or even local symptoms. The treatment of choice is to open the abscess and currette and pack it with bone chips under adequate antibiotic cover; full recovery is almost inevitable.

SEPTIC ARTHRITIS

A primary bacterial infection involving a joint is rare today but staphylococcal septic arthritis is still seen occasionally in neonates and infants with immunologic problems. Tuberculosis, however, involves joints rather than bones now and will be discussed later. A secondary septic arthritis is a well-recognized complication of total joint replacement.

Septic arthritis is often difficult to diagnose radiographically for the first few weeks. The patient will be febrile, complaining of pain, and have limitation of movement in the involved joint. Initially, there may be evidence of a joint effusion (Fig. 4-6A) with displacement of the surrounding fat planes as well as widening of the joint space. At this stage, a bone scan will be strongly positive and an aspiration arthrogram will confirm the diagnosis. As the infection progresses, diffuse bone resorption occurs around the joint producing localized rarefaction radiographically. If the condition still remains untreated, the physeal plate becomes broached and the epiphysis may fall off into the joint capsule (Fig. 4-6B) or even migrate or be totally resorbed (Fig. 4-6C). It is now rare to see this complication in countries with adequate medical facilities. The final result of an untreated septic arthritis is ankylosis which is classically fibrous following bacterial infections and osseous in tuberculosis but in fact either may occur as a sequel to either type of infection.

TUBERCULOSIS

Many people seem to be under the impression that tuberculosis has almost died out, yet this is not the case. In a busy university hospital of 700 beds, we see about 30 new cases of pulmonary tuberculosis per year and about 10 or 12 cases of tuberculous involvement of the musculoskeletal system. Tuberculous osteomyelitis is very rare and was only seen in young children who developed a dactylitis ("spina ventosa") which resembles the bone changes seen in sarcoidosis or brown tumors involving the phalanges. The most common form of tuberculosis seen orthopedically is a tuberculous "septic arthritis" or more correctly a tuberculous synovitis. This is exemplified by tuberculous involvement of the knee where erosions occur at all of the synovial insertions such as the edges of the articular surfaces of the femur and tibia as well as at the insertion of the synovium overlying the cruciates (Fig. 4-7). In North America and Europe, tuberculosis may involve any joint although it seems to have a predilection for the spine, knee, sacroiliac joint, and wrist. Spinal tuberculosis is dealt with under spinal infections.

The patient often presents with swelling and pain in the joint of several weeks duration and has apparently normal x-rays (Fig. 4-8A). If the symptoms persist, a repeat x-ray 1 to 2 months later will show soft tissue swelling and widespread rarefaction (Fig. 4-8B), but no specific erosions or articular joint space changes can be seen. If the diagnosis is still not made, then a repeat radiograph several months later will demonstrate the characteristic erosions as well as loss of joint cartilage space (Fig. 4-8C). Thus, although the appearances of septic arthritis due to bacterial infections and due to tuberculosis are similar, it is the time factor that differs, weeks for bacterial infections and months for tuberculosis. Tuberculous involvement of the sacroiliac joint is usually on the right side, presumably as a result of direct drainage from involved mesenteric lymph nodes. The appearances are of a long-standing abscess with patchy lucent areas and a sclerotic outer margin (Fig. 4-9).

SPINAL INFECTIONS

Spinal infections are most common in the lumbar region, presumably as a result of drainage from infected kidneys or lymphatic drainage from the pelvis and bowel. Traditionally, it has always been taught that in the spine, bacteria involve the bodies of the vertebra producing anterior erosions with marked sclerosis (Fig. 4-10); whereas tuberculosis of the spine involves the disc with destruction of the end plates, rarefaction of the bodies, and no sclerosis (Fig. 4-11). Unfortunately, it has become very difficult to separate the two types of infections on radiographic grounds alone although clinically bacterial infections present with a shorter history and the patient usually has more in the way of systemic symptoms. It is also true that in untreated bacterial infections the vertebral bodies are predominantly involved, leading ultimately to their collapse with relative preservation of the disc space. Classically, in tuberculosis of the spine, however, the disc spaces are lost, and there is anterior wedging of the bodies leading to the classical "gibbus" or acute bend that was frequently seen in the old days (Fig. 4-11B). The majority of bacterial infections of the spine are still caused by staphylococci, although unusual infections may occur in patients who are immunosuppressed (i.e., dialysis or transplant patients) who may get infections with such organisms as *E. coli* and *Pseudomonas*.

OTHER INFECTIONS

SICKLE CELL ANEMIA.   Patients with sickle cell anemia are more prone to get osteomyelitis than normal patients and although *Staphyloccocus aureus* is still the most common organism, salmonella osteomyelitis is not uncommon in these patients. This has a somewhat longer time course than other bacterial infections although the radiographic appearances are similar. Salmonella involvement of the sacroiliac joints resembles tuberculosis, and involvement of the spine may lead to dense vertebral body sclerosis, a so-called ivory vertebra (see the differential diagnosis in Chap. 1).

SYPHILIS.   Syphilis of bone has three classic radiographic manifestations, all of which are extremely rare today: (1) congenital syphilis often leads to a stillborn child with a widespread periosteal reaction on all long bones. (2) Juvenile syphilis may present as a dactylitis similar to tuberculosis. (3) Adult syphilis can present as a gumma which is a localized destructive lesion often of the nasal septum or skull.

GONOCOCCAL ARTHRITIS.   Gonoccal arthritis usually has no radiographic features, but if the infection is allowed to continue untreated, gonococci produce hyaluronidase which destroys articular cartilage and hence produces marked narrowing of the joint space. This occurs usually without underlying osseous changes.

ATYPICAL MYCOBACTERIA AND FUNGI.   Atypical mycobacteria and fungi produce radiographic appearances not unlike chronic osteomyelitis or of tuberculosis. Some fungi, in fact, produce synovial hypertrophy indistinguishable from tuberculosis of the knee, for example.

SCLEROSING OSTEOMYELITIS OF GARRE. Sclerosing osteomyelitis of Garre is said to be a form of chronic osteomyelitis in which part or all of a long bone becomes dense and sclerotic. There is rarely, if ever, however, any evidence that the sclerosis was actually caused by an infection.

REFERENCES

Kemp H: Tuberculosis of the spine. Br J Hosp Med 9:39–48, 1976

Waldvogel FA, Medoff G, Swartz MN: Osteomyelitis: A review of clinical features, therapeutic considerations and unusual aspects (three parts). New Engl J Med 282:198–206, 260–266, 315–322, 1970

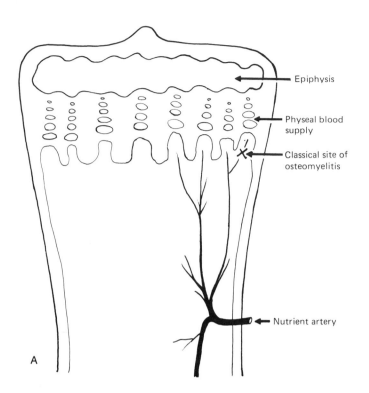

Epiphysis

Physeal blood
supply

Classical site of
osteomyelitis

Nutrient artery

A

FIGURE 4-1: *The pathogenesis of long bone osteomyelitis.* **A.** This drawing illustrates the common site of osteomyelitis in the metaphyseal end of a long bone between the blood supply to the physeal plate and the major diaphyseal nutrient artery supply. **B.** As the infection progresses, the pus runs down between the periosteum and the cortex producing a periosteal reaction (involucrum). The infection also runs down the inside of the cortex often cutting off the blood supply leading to a sequestrum.

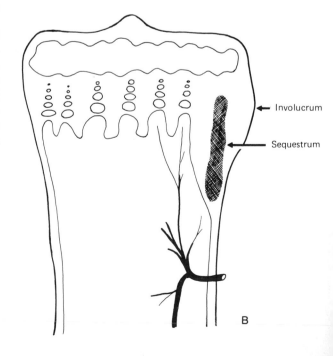

Involucrum

Sequestrum

B

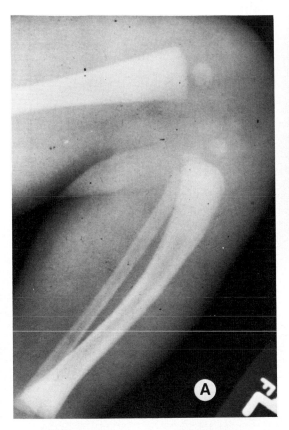

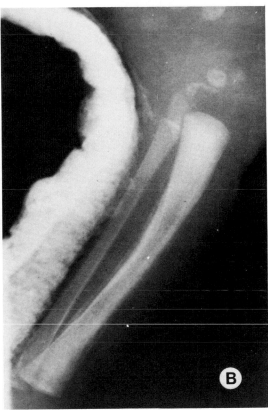

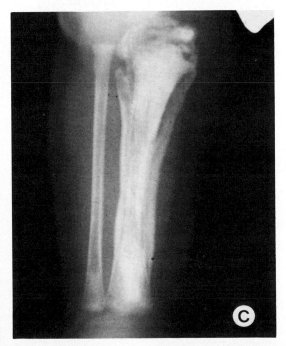

FIGURE 4-2. *Classical bacterial osteomyelitis of the tibia.* **A.** The initial film shows soft tissue swelling and loss of the normal fat planes. **B.** Two weeks later, there is a marked periosteal reaction and the proximal metaphysis of the tibia has become dense. **C.** Two weeks later, the tibia is dense and irregular (sequestrum) and surrounded by marked periosteal new bone (involucrum).

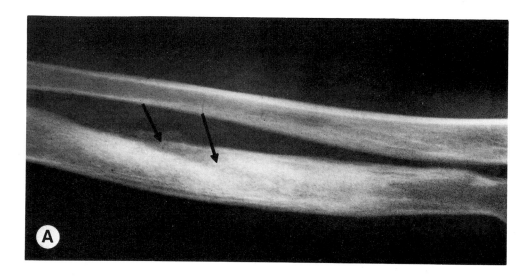

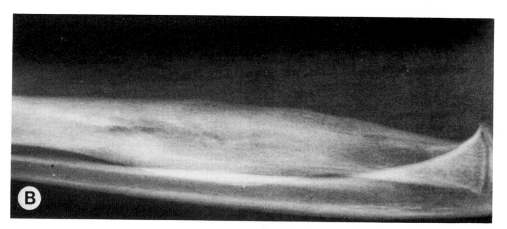

FIGURE 4-3. *Chronic osteomyelitis.*   **A.** AP. **B.** Lateral views. These show a central lucency surrounded by plentiful periosteal new bone with at least one sinus tract or lacuna (arrows) in this 9-year-old boy with chronic osteomyelitis of the right radius.

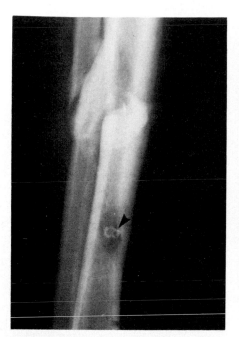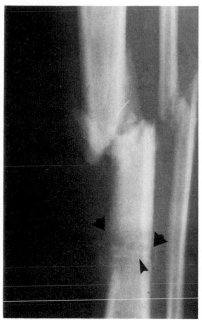

FIGURE 4-4. *Ring sequestrum.*   Following a skiing injury one year previously, these oblique fractures of the tibia and fibula were treated by internal fixation. One of the screws led to an infection and the plate was removed. A sequestrum (small arrows) and an involucrum may be clearly seen (large arrows).

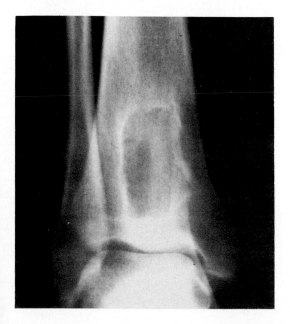

FIGURE 4-5. *Brodie's abscess.*   There is a well-defined lucency at the lower end of the tibia which can be seen to abut on the physeal plate.

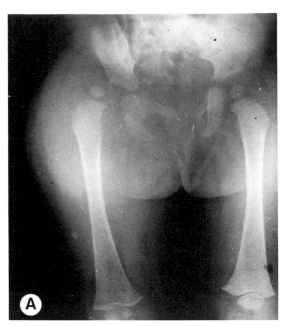

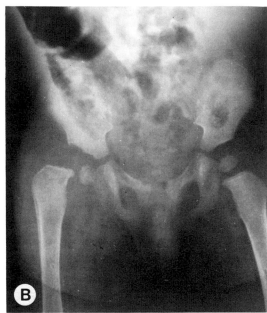

FIGURE 4-6. *Septic arthritis of right hip.* **A.** Initially there is soft tissue swelling and displacement of the right femoral head. **B.** Some days later the femoral head has slipped off and lies within an intact joint capsule. **C.** Several weeks later, the joint capsule has ruptured and the femoral head has been resorbed.

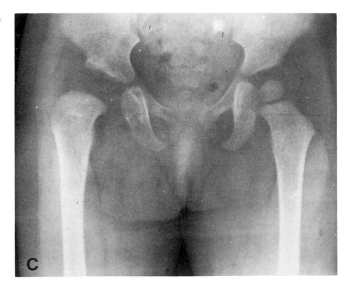

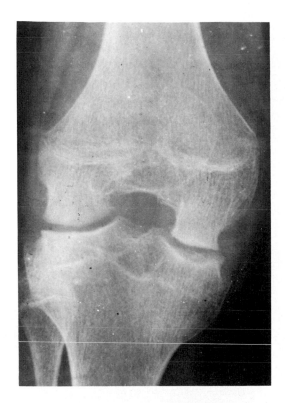

FIGURE 4-7. *Tuberculosis of the knee.* Note the erosions at all the synovial insertions in the knee joint in this young Nigerian male. The intercondylar notch is widened and there are also erosions of the tibial spines. (Reproduced by courtesy of Stanley Bohrer, M.D.)

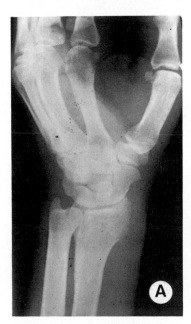
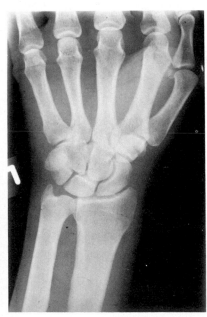

FIGURE 4-8. *Tuberculosis of the wrist.* **A.** Two views of an apparently normal wrist. (For Figs. 4-8B,C see following page.)

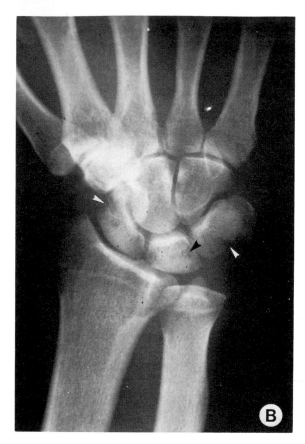

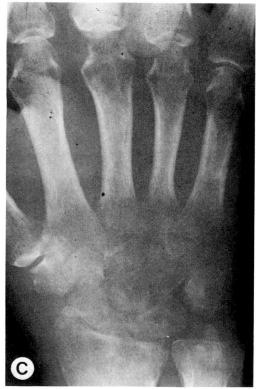

FIGURE 4-8B. One month later discrete erosions are present (arrows) but the joint spaces remain intact. **C.** Four months later there is widespread juxta-articular osteoporosis and multiple erosions as well as obvious loss of joint space in this 49-year-old man with classic tuberculosis of the wrist.

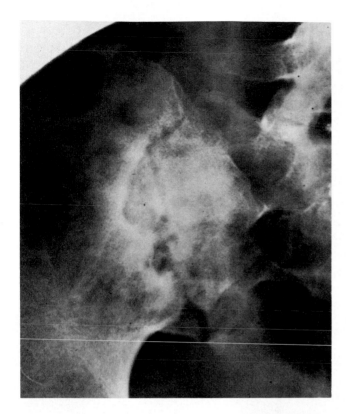

FIGURE 4-9. *Tuberculosis of the right sacroiliac joint.* There are erosions and sclerosis of the right sacroiliac joint with bone destruction and abscess formation in this young female patient with typical pulmonary tuberculosis who was complaining of backache.

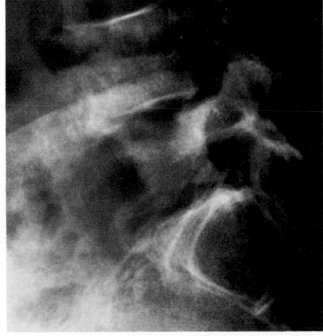

FIGURE 4-10. *Staphylococcal osteomyelitis of the spine.* This unfortunate woman of 51 presented with pain in her back. There is obvious destruction of the anterior surface of both L5 and L4 as well as sclerosis of L5 and narrowing of the L4–5 and L5–S1 disc spaces. At operation, the patient was found to have a huge abscess and staphylococcus osteomyelitis of the spine as well as advanced Hodgkin's disease.

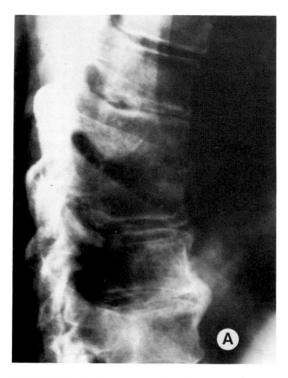

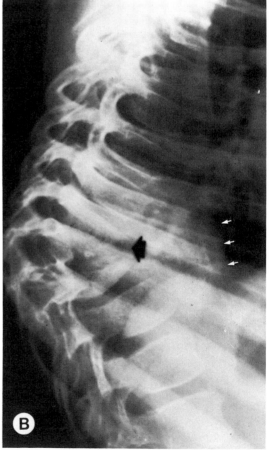

FIGURE 4-11. *Tuberculosis of the spine.* **A.** There is disc space narrowing and destruction of the adjacent end plates in this 68-year-old man with 6-month history of back pain. **B.** In chronic tuberculosis, an acute kyphosis with loss of at least one vertebral body is classical and is known as a "Gibbus" (large arrow). A soft tissue mass is also apparent (small arrows).

FIVE

Metabolic Bone Disease

The term *metabolic bone disease* covers those conditions in which there is some alteration to the metabolism of bone. Bone resorption (from osteoclastic activity) and bone formation (from osteoblastic activity) are equal during adult life, with bone formation being greater than resorption in children and increased resorption occurring in the elderly. But this is not the whole explanation because alterations in the bone matrix have also to be considered as well as the effect of changes in vitamin D intake and the effect of many other chemicals, minerals, and vitamins such as vitamin C, magnesium, zinc, and calcitonin. (These will not be discussed here in detail and the interested reader is referred to the papers and texts listed at the end of Chapter 1.) Before the radiographic features of the important metabolic bone diseases are discussed, it is necessary to briefly consider the various methods of measuring the calcium content of the skeleton.

1. A conventional radiograph demonstrates the morphologic changes present but will only provide us with a rough idea of the true mineral content of the bones.
2. Special standardized films may be taken with or without step wedges and standards, such as the metacarpal bones.
3. Measurements of the amount of cortical bone with respect to cancellous bone may be made such as at the midshaft of the second metacarpal where 45 percent of the bone should be cortical (metacarpal index).

4. Examining a specially taken radiograph with a photodensitometer may be used, but the more accurate methods of bone mineral measurement depend largely on radioactive isotopes.
5. Neutron activation, which is difficult and cumbersome.
6. The use of a photon absorptiometer which is a portable external isotopic point source (^{125}I) capable of scanning a limb to provide a very accurate measurement of calcium content.

Whichever method is used, the bone mineral content is important and will be mentioned for many of the metabolic conditions discussed below.

OSTEOPOROSIS

Classic osteoporosis involves the spine and long bones in elderly patients, but there are many causes of "osteopenia" (Table 5-1). Osteopenia is a better word to use than osteoporosis for the "thin bones" or poorly mineralized bones seen radiographically when the true cause of the loss of bone mineral is unknown. The bone mineral content in men remains fairly constant until the age of 60 whereas in women the bone mineral content rises to a peak at about 35 or 40 after which it begins to fall quite rapidly.

Table 5-1

The Causes of Osteopenia

1. Postmenopausal
2. Senility
3. Hypogonadism and eunuch
4. Cushing's disease
5. Acromegaly
6. Hyperparathyroidism
7. Hyperthyroidism
8. Steroids
9. Fragilitas ossium
10. Immobilization and disuse atrophy
11. Sudeck's atrophy
12. Malnutrition
13. Idiopathic
14. Myelomatosis
15. Diabetes
16. Osteomalacia (see Table 5-2)
17. Malabsorption syndrome
18. Scurvy and decreased vitamin C
19. Heparin therapy
20. Addison's disease
21. Nonendocrine neoplasms

The loss of bone mineral that accompanies aging can be termed senile, or postmenopausal osteoporosis but possibly better terms would be involutional osteoporosis or physiologic bone atrophy. True osteoporosis is a disease where there is a marked increase in bone resorption often in middle-aged females who present with fractures of the wrist or femoral neck. Cancellous bone is resorbed first with accompanying loss of the secondary trabeculae before the primary stress-bearing trabeculae are resorbed and before there is any noticeable loss of cortical bone.

The radiographic features of osteoporosis are as follows:

1. In long bones, there is resorption of the secondary trabeculae and subsequent accentuation of the primary weight-bearing trabeculae as well as eventual thinning of the cortices. This is well seen in the femoral neck (Fig. 5-1).
2. In the vertebral bodies, resorption of the secondary trabeculae followed by resorption of the primary trabeculae causes "pencilling" of the end plates which become very clear cut and more obvious than normal (Fig. 5-2A).
3. Ultimately the disc becomes relatively stronger than the vertebral bodies so that the end plates sag and the so-called fishmouth or codfish vertebral body ensues.
4. Fractures of the vertebral bodies also occur apart from the "codfishing" and many patients experience back pain from microfractures that are histologically, but not radiologically visible. Ultimately severe wedge fractures occur often with complete collapse of one or more vertebral bodies (Fig. 5-2B).
5. Other fractures are common in patients with osteoporosis and classically involve the ends of long bones where there is rapid bone turnover and increased resorption of cancellous bone, i.e., in the femoral necks, distal radius, and proximal humerus.

OSTEOMALACIA

Osteomalacia (and rickets) is caused by an abnormality of vitamin D metabolism (Table 5-2). Although long-standing osteomalacia has a classic radiologic appearance, the radiographic diagnosis of early osteomalacia is more difficult. Subclinical osteomalacia is much more common than was originally thought, particularly in elderly people. The primary defect in osteomalacia is a failure of mineralization of the osteoid so that the bone mineral content may actually be normal but there is increased unmineralized osteoid seen histologically. To use a simplistic analogy, osteoporosis is a disease of bone quantity (i.e., a loss of bone volume) whereas osteomalacia is a disease of bone quality (i.e., the volume remains normal but the amount of mineralized bone decreases).

Table 5-2

Etiology of Osteomalacia

Dietary
1. Vitamin D lack

Intestinal Malabsorption
1. Celiac disease
2. Idiopathic steatorrhea
3. Postgastrectomy
4. Chronic cirrhosis
5. Biliary rickets (congenital biliary obstruction)
6. Inflammatory bowel disease

Renal Diseases
1. Fanconi's syndrome
2. Familial vitamin D-resistant osteomalacia
3. Hyperchloremic renal acidosis
4. Chronic acetozemic renal failure

Other
1. Hypophosphatasemia
2. Anticonvulsant therapy

The radiographic diagnosis of early osteomalacia consists of three elements. (1) *Intracortical tunneling* occurs in long bones and can be seen using high resolution x-ray films (by employing mammographic, industrial, or magnification techniques). These linear intracortical streaks represent increased osteocytic osteoclastic activity (Fig. 5-3), and they are actually widened Haversian canals which may be seen in states of increased bone turnover such as osteomalacia, hyperparathyroidism, thyrotoxicosis, and disuse osteoporosis. (2) A *blurred trabecular pattern* with disordered trabeculae may also be seen in osteomalacia unlike in pure osteoporosis where the individual trabeculum remains clearly defined. (3) There is *blurring of the end plates* and trabeculae in the vertebral bodies in pure osteomalacia unlike in osteoporosis where there is loss of both the primary and secondary trabeculae with penciling of the clear-cut vertebral end plates.

The radiographic diagnosis of classic osteomalacia also consists of three elements. (1) There is *generalized osteopenia* with blurring of the trabeculae. (2) The typical abnormality is a *pseudofracture* (Fig. 5-4A). These are areas of localized loss of mineral although the underlying matrix is intact, at least initially. Pseudofractures occur at points of stress and are often symmetrical. Classically, they may be seen in the pubic and ischial rami, on the under surface of the femoral necks and upper humeri as well as in the upper ribs, scapulae, and long bones. Some of these lucencies have surrounding sclerosis which is due to reactive new bone as an attempt occurs to heal these lesions. These are known as *Looser zones* (Fig. 5-4B). The differential diagnosis of a true fracture from a pseudofracture is simple in that the patient with osteomalacia is usually lethargic with a long history of malabsorption or renal problems and the lesions are painless. (3) Pseudofractures do represent areas of potential weakness, and if the osteomalacia is not promptly treated, then they will become *true fractures*. It is not uncommon to see a slipped capital femoral epiphysis or distortion of the bony pelvis (a "champagne glass" pelvis) with protrusio acetabuli in patients with long-standing untreated osteomalacia.

RICKETS

Rickets is osteomalacia in children. With the growth potential of the physeal plate, the most remarkable radiographic changes occur at this site, and thus are best seen at the major growing epiphyses, such as the distal radius and around the knee. The radiographic appearance of rickets is characteristic with broadening of the physeal plate, widening of the metaphyseal end of the bone, and fraying of its surface with cupping (Fig. 5-5). An abnormal trabecular pattern with coarse blurred trabeculae is often also seen as it is in adult osteomalacia.

SCURVY

Pure lack of vitamin C is now only seen in people who are deprived of adequate fresh fruit either due to religious reasons or poor diet. In adults, the clinical manifestations of scurvy usually present before a generalized periosteal reaction becomes apparent radiologically. The patient will have bleeding gums and petechiae which are due to increased capillary fragility because vitamin C is required for a number of stages in collagen synthesis and also for adequate mineralization of the skeleton.

The radiographic appearance of scurvy in children includes widened metaphyses with accentuation of the adjacent metaphyseal plate which has a lucency underlying it (Fig. 5-6). This represents a point of weakness and fractures occur here with subsequent slippage of the physeal plate and adjacent metaphysis. The epiphysis has a lucency ("ring sign") under its subchondral margins which, similar to the lucency in the metaphysis, is due to a failure of mineralization in the provisional zone of calcification.

HYPERPARATHYROIDISM

This may be either primary (due to an adenoma or hyperplasia of the parathyroid glands) or secondary (due to renal failure and the ensuing abnormalities in calcium/phosphate metabolism). In either case, the changes may be identical although osteosclerosis is more common in patients with secondary hyperparathyroidism. The elevated parathyroid hormone stimulates osteoclasts to resorb excess bone which is replaced by fibrous tissue, hence the old name "osteitis fibrosa et cystica." This may be localized (cysts or "brown tumors") or generalized. The excess calcium may be deposited in soft tissues, blood vessels, or specific organs such as the kidneys where it may be seen as nephrocalcinosis. Clinically the patient complains of weakness, polyuria, polydipsia, anorexia, nausea, vomiting, as well as bone pain. Mental confusion may also occur.

The radiographic changes of hyperparathyroidism include:

1. *Osteoporosis:* generalized osteoporosis with spontaneous or stress fractures, cortical bone resorption, trabecular bone resorption, and subperiosteal bone resorption which is pathognomonic of hyperparathyroidism and is best seen on the radial aspect of the middle phalanx of the second and third fingers as well as in the tufts of the fingers (Fig. 5-7A).
2. *Localized cysts* may occur: brown tumors (Fig. 5-7B) which represent localized areas of resorption into which there has been bleeding, hence the term *brown.* They are not true tumors. Von Recklinghausen's disease (osteitis fibrosa et cystica) represents a more generalized form of this condition. Note that in spite of what the older literature implies giant cell tumors are rare in hyperparathyroidism.
3. *In the skull,* there are scattered areas of demineralization and osteosclerosis producing a so-called "salt and pepper" skull.
4. *Osteosclerosis:* sclerotic bands may be seen adjacent to the end plates of the vertebral bodies ("Rugger Jersey spine") and are more common in renal failure than in primary hyperparathyroidism (Fig. 5-7C); generalized osteosclerosis may also be seen in both primary and secondary hyperparathyroidism.
5. *Localized resorption* occurs at certain sites but particularly at the acromioclavicular joints; sacroiliac joints and symphysis pubis and these changes are also commonly seen in both primary and secondary hyperparathyroidism (Fig. 5-7D).
6. *The bone mineral content* is markedly decreased, and this can be corrected by parathyroidectomy in patients with primary hyper-

parathyroidism but is more difficult to correct in patients with secondary disease.

RENAL BONE DISEASE

The initial descriptions of the bone disease seen in renal failure ("renal osteodystrophy") implied that it was mainly due to hyperparathyroidism, but in fact osteoporosis and osteomalacia also occur commonly in these patients. In a recent histologic study, in fact, 95 percent of dialysis patients had histologic evidence of osteomalacia, 60 percent had evidence of hyperparathyroidism, and about 20 percent showed some loss of trabecular bone (osteoporosis). In 100 long-term renal dialysis patients, we were able to radiologically demonstrate hyperparathyroidism in 50 percent, osteomalacia in 20 percent, and osteosclerosis in 20 percent. Photon absorptiometry revealed a significant loss of bone mineral content in 75 percent of the patients.

HYPOPARATHYROIDISM

This condition is rare and has few radiographic features although calcification of the basal ganglia, premature closure of the epiphyses, and sclerosis of the physeal plates and vertebral end plates have been described.

ACROMEGALY

Acromegaly is due to an eosinophilic pituitary adenoma which produces excess growth hormone. If this situation occurs before the epiphyses fuse, the result is a giant. But acromegaly is more frequent in adults and anything which can still grow does so. This includes bone at muscle origins, in the metaphyseal regions of long bones where there is no periosteum, the articular cartilage, and the soft tissues. The clinical features of acromegaly include overgrowth of the hands, feet, skull, scalp, and tongue.

The radiographic features of acromegaly are many:

1. In the *hand*, there is increased thickening of the tufts, metacarpals, and sites of muscle origin as well as increasing soft tissue thickness and joint cartilage widening. This produces a "spadelike" hand (Fig. 5-8A).

2. In the *skull*, there is increased thickness of the skull tables with enlargement of the frontal sinuses, elongation of the mandible with increasing prominence (prognathism), and separation of the teeth which leads to decay and ultimately to an edentulous patient. Also, the sella turcica is increased in size by the tumor, often with erosion of the clinoids (Fig. 5-8B).

3. In the *heel pad*, the normal thickness of the heel pad is up to 21 mm from the lowest point of the os calcis to the edge of the soft tissues measured vertically (Fig. 5-8C). Most acromegalics have a heel pad thickness greater than 25 mm; but be careful to exclude normal patients who have calluses on their feet or those with congestive cardiac failure or myxedema.

4. In the *vertebral bodies*, the thoracic spine has increased new bone anteriorly whereas there is increasing concavity of the posterior surfaces in the lumbar region due to overgrowth of the meninges (Fig. 5-8D).

5. *Soft tissue enlargement.* There is obvious enlargement in soft tissue thickness not only in the hands, feet, heel pad, and tongue but also in the viscera and the heart.

6. In the *joints*, there is apparent increase in joint space width, but, in fact, it is fibrocartilage replacing hyaline cartilage and thus premature degenerative arthritis occurs rapidly primarily in the weight-bearing joints (Fig. 5-8E).

PRIMARY AND SECONDARY CUSHING'S DISEASE

Primary Cushing's disease is rare and occurs as a result of overactivity of the adrenal glands due to either hyperplasia or a tumor such as an adrenal carcinoma. Occasionally Cushing's disease may be due to a pituitary chromophobe adenoma. Secondary Cushing's disease is much more common and is the result of long-term steroid therapy such as is seen in patients with asthma, lupus erythematosus, and ulcerative colitis. Clinically the patients appear "Cushingoid" and have fat bodies and thin legs ("a lemon on toothpicks"), a dowagers hump, hypertension, and a "moon" facies.

The radiographic features of Cushing's disease include severe osteoporosis that mainly involves the spine and axial skeleton, and in fact the bone mineral content of the limbs is usually normal. "Codfish" vertebrae, vertebral wedging and collapse are common (Fig. 5-9A,B). The callus in fractures of the pelvis, ribs, and long bones has a characteristic appearance: it is exuberant and disorganized ("cotton wool") (Fig. 5-9C). Avascular necrosis also occurs frequently and is most often seen in the femoral or humeral head (Fig. 5-9D). Note also that repeated intra-articular injections of steroids leads to joint destruction and neuropathic joints.

PAGET'S DISEASE

Although this is not a true metabolic disease, Paget's disease appears to be due to an imbalance of osteoclastic and osteoblastic activity which may be metabolic in origin. It was first described by Sir James Paget in 1877. The etiology of Paget's disease is unknown but it is very rare in patients under 50. It appears to be more common in northern climates such as that in Finland and Canada and gets rarer the further south one goes so that it is never seen in Egypt and the Caribbean. It is often found serendipidously. Paget's disease may be monosteal or generalized, and pathologically there is increased resorption with disorganization of bone and a characteristic "mosaic" pattern histologically. The resorption is rapidly followed by new bone formation and in most mature forms of Paget's disease the equilibrium between resorption and new bone formation seems to have been regained. The alkaline phosphatase is markedly elevated in most patients with active Paget's disease.

The radiographic features of Paget's disease are very characteristic: The involved bone may show increased lucency or increased sclerosis or both. In long bones initially Paget's disease is associated with increased osteoclasis and hence there is an increased risk of pathologic fractures. There is extensive remodeling in Paget's disease with some classic features including:

1. Actual expansion of the involved bone.
2. Thickening of the cortex particularly in the pelvis where the iliopectineal line is thickened in 90 percent of cases of Paget's disease (Fig. 5-10A).
3. Deformities also can occur such as microfractures as well as true fractures and bowing of long bones and protrusio acetabulae of the hips.
4. There is an abnormal trabecular pattern in Paget's disease with patchy areas of lucency (Fig. 5-10B) and of sclerosis associated with large irregular trabeculae.
5. Incremental fractures of long bones occur on the convexity of the curvature (Fig. 5-10C).
6. A "candle flame" lucency may be the first stage of Paget's disease of a long bone which is often best seen at the end of the femur or in the midshaft of the tibia (Fig. 5-10D).

There are a number of specific complications to Paget's disease and these include pain in the involved bone, fractures often through a lucent area of the "candle flame," cardiac failure due to increased vascularity, and deafness and headaches if the skull is involved. Malignant change into a sarcoma (usually an osteosarcoma) is actually rare but does occur. There are a number of specific treatments for Paget's disease: calcitonin, mithramycin, and diphosphonates may relieve the pain and arrest (rather than cure) the disease.

The differential diagnosis of the radiographic features of Paget's disease include osteoblastic metastases (but these do not usually widen the bone), Hodgkin's disease (which occurs in younger patients and is not generally so widespread), hyperparathyroidism (but subperiosteal erosions do not occur in Paget's disease), and fluorosis.

THYROID BONE DISEASE

Most patients with hyperthyroidism or cretinism and myxedema are treated before any skeletal changes manifest themselves. In thyrotoxicosis, however, occasionally a profound osteopenia becomes apparent and intracortical tunneling may be seen in the phalanges. Cretinism produces a severe retardation of skeletal maturity (Fig. 5-11) as well as a generalized increase in bone density. Finally, there is a rare form of perpendicular periosteal reaction involving the metacarpals and phalanges which occurs in some patients who become myxedematous following ablation of the thyroid gland for severe thyrotoxicosis. This is known as thyroid acropachy.

REFERENCES

See Chapter 1 for references on bone morphology.

Renal Bone Disease

Griffiths HJ: The Radiology of Renal Failure. Philadelphia, Saunders, 1976

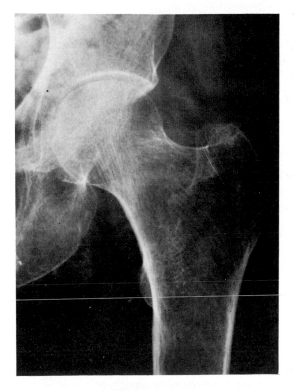

FIGURE 5-1. *Osteoporosis—Femoral Neck.* This 80-year-old woman is complaining of pain in the region of the left hip. She is seen to be "osteopenic" with loss of cortical thickness and secondary trabeculae as well as a thinning of the few remaining primary trabeculae.

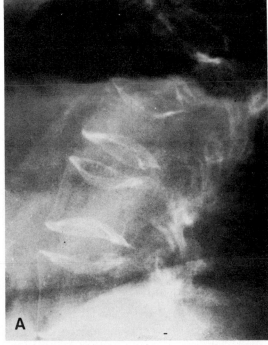

FIGURE 5-2. *Osteoporosis—Spine.* **A.** Lumbo-sacral spine, with moderate osteoporosis. The apparent increased whiteness ("penciling") can be seen in the vertebral end plates which are biconcave (the so-called codfish or fishmouth vertebrae). This appearance is due to the loss of secondary trabeculae within the vertebral body itself thus leading to relative weakness of the body allowing the disc apparently to expand. (For Fig. 5-2B see following page.)

FIGURE 5-2B. *The thoracic spine, in advanced osteoporosis.* This 72-year-old woman has many vertebral bodies wedged or actually collapsing. The increase in density within some of the bodies may be due to actual impaction of bone fragments or to callus formation in association with attempted healing of a previous fracture. Thus, it is often difficult to accurately assess the age of a compression fracture in an osteoporotic patient.

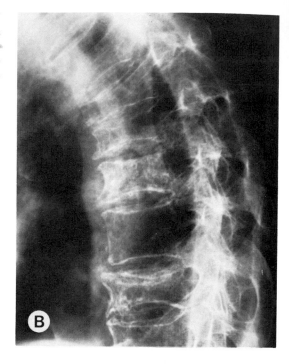

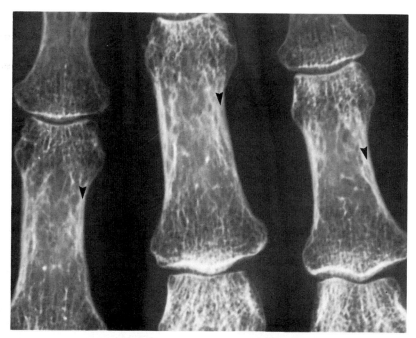

FIGURE 5-3. *Early Osteomalacia.* This 53-year-old woman has nutritional osteomalacia. Although there is generalized loss of bone, the pathognomonic sign is the intracortical tunneling (arrows) which is only seen in states of rapid bone turnover.

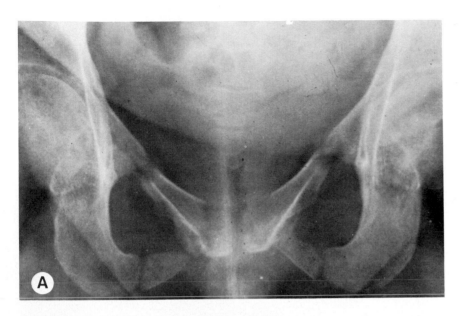

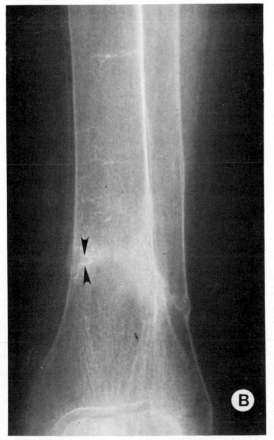

FIGURE 5-4. *Advanced Osteomalacia.* **A.** Pelvis. This 41-year-old missionary suffers from malabsorption syndrome and had long-standing osteomalacia. Note the symmetrical lucencies running at right angles to the edges of the pubic and ischial rami. These are typical of pseudofractures. **B.** Lower tibia and fibula. In a different patient with severe osteomalacia, note the generalized osteopenia, as well as the transverse defect with sclerotic margins (arrows) which represents a Looser zone. This is continuous with a sclerotic area in both the tibia and fibula that represents a pseudofracture that has undergone a true fracture and impacted.

FIGURE 5-5. *Rickets.* There is fraying, irregularity, and widening of the physeal plate in this 4-year-old child with rickets. There is also delay in skeletal maturation as well as an irregular trabecular pattern well seen in the metacarpals.

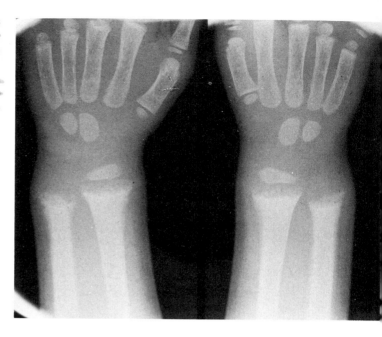

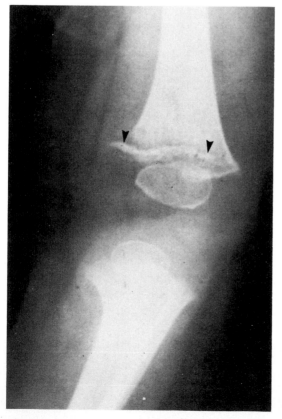

- Metaphyseal spelazing
- Trummerfeld zone (↑ fragmentation)
- white line of Fraenkel (persistent zone of calcification)
- Pelkan Beak (lifted periosteum)
- Wimberger's Ring Sign

FIGURE 5-6. *Scurvy.* Although there is some widening of the physeal plate, the most obvious change is a lucency under the metaphyseal part of the juxtaphyseal bone which has in fact fractured and slipped off (arrows). The epiphysis is noted to show increased density around the edge but a specific lucency underlying this region cannot be seen in this case.

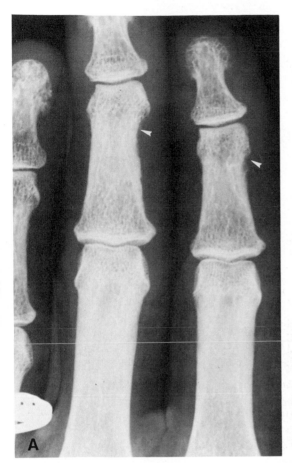

FIGURE 5-7. *Hyperparathyroidism.* **A.** Subperiosteal erosions (arrows) on the radial aspect of the middle phalanges of the second and third fingers is a pathognomonic sign of hyperparathyroidism. Note the disorganized trabecular pattern and the presence of intracortical tunneling.

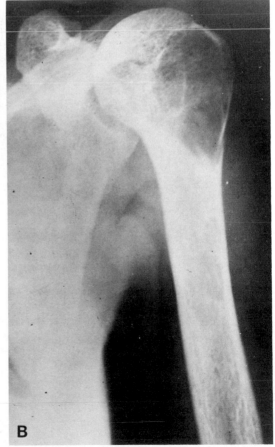

FIGURE 5-7B. Brown tumors in the upper humerus. This large metaphyseal lucency is typical of a brown tumor. (For Figs. 5-7C, D see following page.)

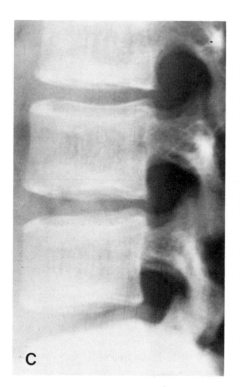

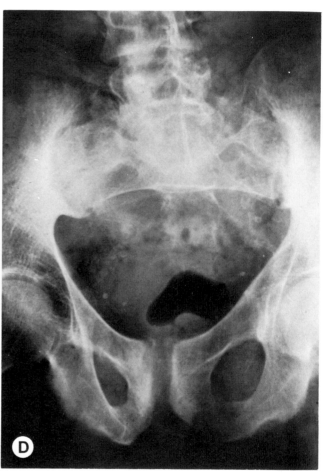

FIGURE 5-7C. Rugger jersey spine. The increased density adjacent to the vertebral end plates with relative sparing of the central part of the vertebral body is typically seen in renal bone disease (secondary hyperparathyroidism). **D.** Pelvis. Localized resorption at the sacroiliac joints with widening of the sacroiliac joint, sclerosis of the iliac border and with a disorganized trabecular pattern as well as widening and irregularity of the symphysis pubis is typical of hyperparathyroidism.

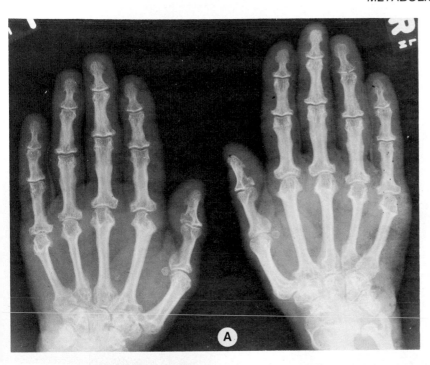

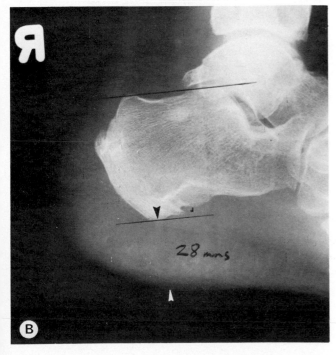

FIGURE 5-8. *Acromegaly.*   **A.** Hands. There is an overgrowth of bone in the metaphyseal regions particularly of the radius, ulna, and metacarpal heads. There is enlargement of the soft tissues (spadelike hand) and some widening of some of the joint spaces. **B.** Heel pad. In a normal person, the thickness of the heel pad measured between the most dependent part of the calcaneum and a perpendicular line drawn to the skin (arrows) should be below 21 mm. In most acromegalics, this measurement is above 25 mm. (For Figs. 5-8C,D,E see following pages.)

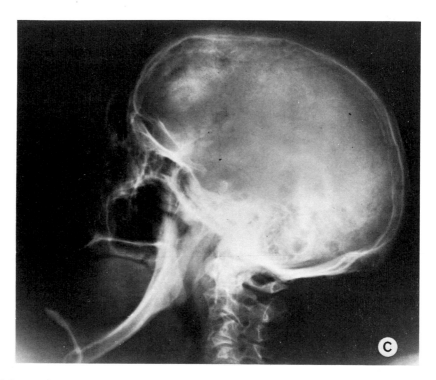

FIGURE 5-8 continued.   C. Skull. There is thickening of the calvarium with enlargement of the frontal sinuses and prominence of the occipital protuberance. The jaw has elongated and lost its normal angulation. Note that the patient has become edentulous and is suffering from macroglossia. There is also enlargement of the sella turcica. **D.** Spine. There is scalloping of the posterior aspect of the lumbar vertical bodies due to enlargement of the theca and pressure erosion. Conversely new bone is laid down anteriorly on the thoracic vertebral bodies (arrow). **E.** Pelvis. Severe premature osteoarthritis with loss of the joint cartilage space and (acromegalic) osteophyte formation has occurred in this 50-year-old patient with long-standing acromegaly.

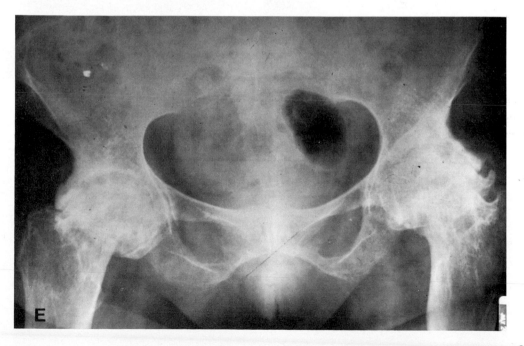

FIGURE 5-8, continued.

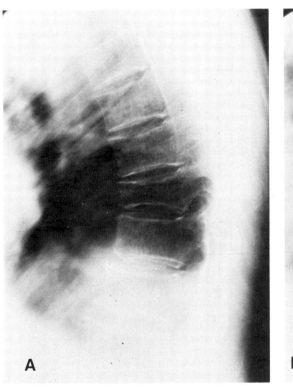

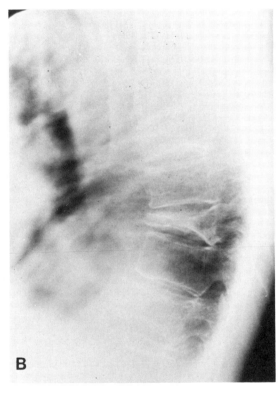

A

B

FIGURE 5-9. *Cushing's Disease (Primary and Secondary).*   **A,B.** This 42-year-old woman was on steroid therapy for asthma and continued to take ever increasing doses of steroids despite warnings of the danger of osteoporosis. **A.** Film of 7/9/68 shows osteopenia with some compression fractures. **B.** Film of 3/5/69 shows further compression and more advanced demineralization (compare to Fig. 5-1). **C.** Cotton wool callus formation. This 52-year-old man was receiving steroid therapy for systemic lupus erythematosus. He sus- tained a Colles fracture and this is the appearance 6 weeks later in spite of adequate immobilization. **D.** Avascular necrosis in Cushing's disease. This middle-aged man presented with obesity and pain in both hips. The radiograph shows bilateral in- crease in density in both femoral heads with some collapse of the left side. He was found to have Cushing's disease and both femoral heads dem- onstrated the classic changes of avascular nec- rosis pathologically. (For Figs. 5-9C,D see facing page.)

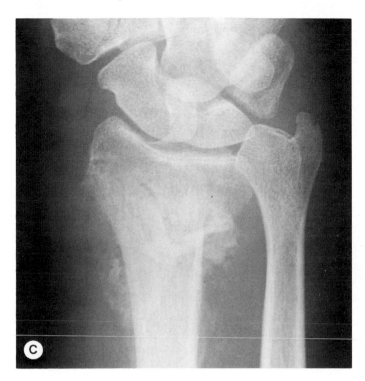

FIGURE 5-9, continued

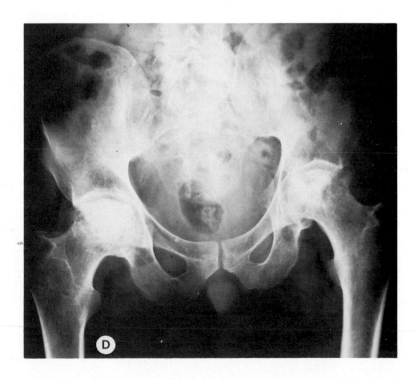

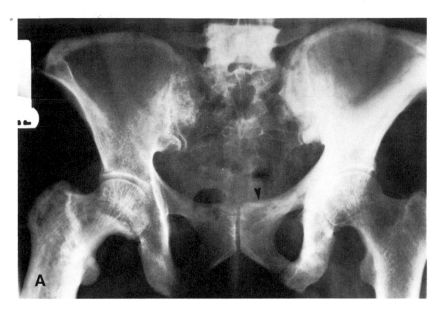

FIGURE 5-10. *Paget's Disease.* **A.** Pelvis. There is thickening, and increased bone density and a disorganized trabecular pattern seen in the left half of the pelvis, right femur and in L5 ("ivory vertebrae"). Note the thickening of the iliopectineal line on the left (arrow).

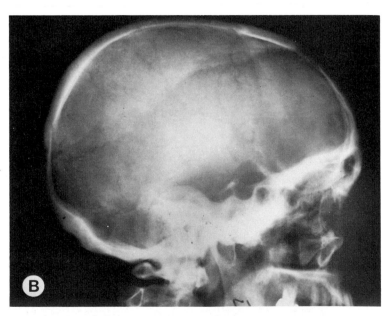

basal index > 160
⇒ basilar invagination
- petroclinoid lig. calcification
- flattening of occiput
- Cotton wool

FIGURE 5-10B. *Skull.* There is a well-circumscribed bandlike lucency running around the skull which is typical of osteoporosis circumscripta seen in early Paget's disease of the skull. (For Figs. 5-10C,D see facing page.)

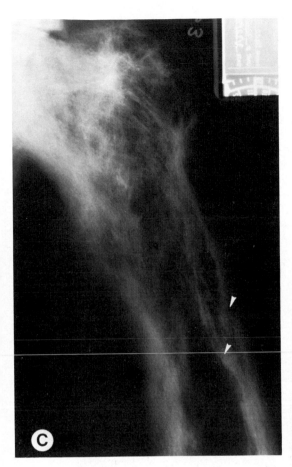

FIGURE 5-10C. *Incremental fractures.* In this 58-year-old woman with Paget's disease of the left femur, there are a number of horizontal lines (arrows) which represent incremental fractures.

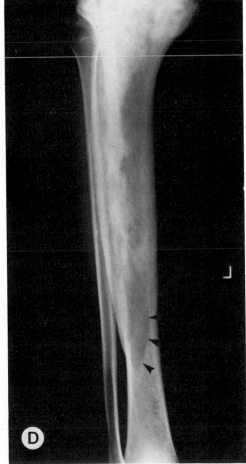

Blade of grass

FIGURE 5-10D. *Tibia.* There is a "candle flame lucency" (arrows) in the distal tibia. This represents the advancing front of the Paget's disease.

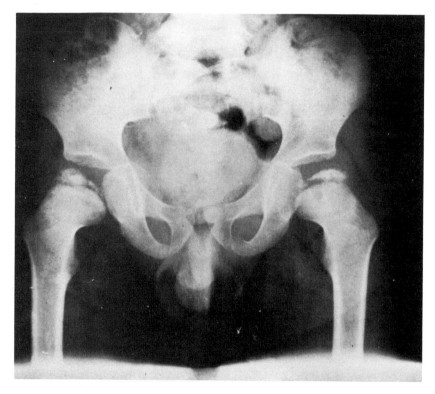

FIGURE 5-11. *Cretinism.*   This 9-year-old child has retarded bone age, fragmentation, and deformity of both femoral heads as well as widening and distortion of the metaphyseal regions of the femoral necks, all of which are typical findings in cretinism.

SIX

Arthritis

Although we use the term *arthritis* in general, there are several main types of arthritis including degenerative arthritis, rheumatoid arthritis (and its variants), and gout. It is possible for the radiologist to make the correct diagnosis in over 95 percent of patients with arthritis if a number of clinical facts, biochemical data, and the radiologic features of the case are known. The *age* and *sex* of the patient are important (Table 6-1); as is the *distribution* of the arthritis, both with respect to the *types of joints* involved and to the *symmetry* of the disease (Table 6-2). If one of the rheumatoid variants is suspected then certain *biochemical data* are important, such as whether the rheumatoid factor and the HLA B27* are positive or not (Table 6-3).

The radiographic features of each type of arthritis will be dealt with individually. In general, however, it is important to look for *soft tissue swelling* (generalized or localized); *calcifications* either in the soft tissues (tophi) or in the joint cartilage (chondrocalcinosis); changes in the *joint cartilage space* (and remember, for instance, always to take AP weight-bearing views of the knees); and effusions and see if the joint space is narrowed. Search for *reactive changes*, for instance, sclerosis and osteophytes in degenerative arthritis, or is there evidence of juxta-articular *osteoporosis* and *erosions* that would suggest rheumatoid arthritis? Look to see if the *erosions* or *cysts* have clear-cut margins (degenerative arthritis and gout) or no apparent edge (rheumatoid arthritis), and to see if they

*HLA B27 refers to a specific antigen on the gene of the sixth chromosome which appears to influence resistance or susceptibility to certain diseases such as ankylosing spondylitis and Reiter's syndromes.

are related to the joint (degenerative arthritis) or even appear to be away from it (gout). If the patient presents with pain in the back, analyze the radiographs to see if there is evidence of a *slipped disc* or *sacroiliitis*. If *sacroiliitis* is present, find out if it is bilateral and symmetrical and associated with erosions, blurring of the margins, and sclerosis which would suggest ankylosing spondylitis; or look to see if the sacroiliitis is not symmetrical, but is still associated with erosions of the sacroiliac joints and irregularity of the apophyseal joints, which suggests either psoriatic or enteropathic arthritis.

This gives you an idea of the kind of intellectual approach that is necessary in order to diagnose an "unknown" case of arthritis. I will now consider each type of arthritis separately, but before the description begins, review Tables 6-1, 6-2, and 6-3 to put these conditions into perspective.

OSTEOARTHRITIS OR DEGENERATIVE ARTHRITIS

The terms *degenerative arthritis* and *osteoarthritis* are interchangeable and refer to one common specific type of arthritis. Degenerative arthritis occurs in older people of both sexes and involves predominantly the weight-bearing joints such as the hips and the knees. It is usually bilateral but not really symmetrical. Osteoarthritis may involve any joint but is frequently seen in the knees, hips, spine, shoulders, ankles, and hands. The classic description of osteoarthritis in the hands is of involvement of the distal interphalangeal joints with small bursae overlying the osteophytes which are known as *Heberden's nodes* (after William Heberden who was an 18th-century English physician and botanist). The first carpometacarpal joint is the joint most frequently involved by osteoarthritis in the upper extremity. Incidentally, if osteophytes (and their accompanying bursae) occur at the proximal interphalangeal joints, they are known as *Bouchard's nodes,* after Charles Jacques Bouchard (1837–1915).

Clinically the patient will complain of pain and increasing difficulty in movement of the affected joint. There will also be recurrent swelling (effusions) and increasing deformity. The rheumatoid factor and HLA B27 are both negative.

Radiographically the characteristic changes are narrowing of the joint space with associated hypertrophic changes, including subchondral sclerosis and osteophyte formation at the edges of the affected joint (Fig. 6-1). The osteophytes can break off and become loose bodies. As this degenerative process continues, the joint space may become totally obliterated. This is associated with a raised intracapsular pressure and small infractions occur through the subchondral bone which is now almost totally denuded of cartilage. This process is known as *eburnation.* Synovial

Table 6-1

Age and Sex of Patients with Arthritis

Disease	Age (yrs)	Sex
JRA	Young	Either male or female
AS	20	Male
Reiter's	20–30	Male
RA	30	Female
Psoriatic	40	Either male or female
Gout	40–50	Predominantly male
Pseudogout	50	Female
OA	50 and older	Either male or female
Collagen	Any age	Female

Table 6-2

The Distribution and Symmetry of Joints Involved with Arthritis

Symmetry	Distribution
RA (most symmetrical)	RA (Smallest joints)
Pseudogout	Variants—Psoriatic
AS/Reiter's	Collagen diseases
OA	Gout
Psoriatic	Pseudogout
JRA	AS and Reiter's
Gout (most asymmetrical)	OA (largest joints)

Table 6-3

The Relationship Between HLA B27 and Arthritis

Ankylosing spondylitis	90–100%
Reiter's syndrome	65–95%
Psoriatic spondylitis	60–100%
Enteropathic spondylitis	70–75%
Yersinia arthritis	90%
JRA	40%
RA	6%
Normal population	4–8%

fluid is forced through these cracks to form subchondral cysts or *geodes* which comes from an old French term meaning a hollow cavity (Fig. 6-2). Geodes are usually seen on both sides of an affected joint and have obvious sclerotic margins. They are most commonly seen in the hip joints where they may give the orthopedist problems during a total hip replacement. Incidentally, there is a high incidence of avascular necrosis in association with degenerative arthritis particularly of the hip.

Varieties of Degenerative Arthritis

SECONDARY OSTEOARTHRITIS.   Secondary osteoarthritis may occur as a result of a previous fracture or dislocation, but it also may be secondary to a previous infection or as a result of abnormal stress placed on a joint such as is seen in genu valgus or in slipped capital femoral epiphysis (Fig. 6-3, see Chap. 9). The radiographic appearances are identical to that seen in primary osteoarthritis, but the diagnosis of secondary osteoarthritis should be kept in mind in younger patients presenting with degenerative changes in a solitary joint. The clinical history (of septic arthritis, dislocation, or fracture involving a joint) as well as the radiographic appearance should provide a clue as to the underlying disorder.

EROSIVE OSTEOARTHRITIS.   There is another form of degenerative arthritis in which erosions can be seen at the joint margins rather than the more centrally placed subchondral cysts. These erosive changes are associated with rapid onset clinically, an inflammatory reaction of the synovium, and marked eburnation of the joint cartilage. Erosive osteoarthritis is seen most frequently in the small joints of the fingers and hands, although it can occur in other joints such as the knees and feet.

FORRESTIER'S DISEASE (DISH—DISSEMINATED IDIOPATHIC SKELETAL HYPEROSTOSIS.   Forrestier first described this common form of acute inflammatory osteoarthritis which involves the spine and major joints in 1949. It appears to have a more rapid onset than typical osteoarthritis; it seems to occur in younger people and is associated with exacerbations of pain and swelling, followed by remissions, thus differentiating it from the more chronic protracted course of classic degenerative arthritis.

The unique radiographic appearance of Forrestier's disease includes the presence of large "osteophytes" which may actually bridge around the joint, particularly in the spine (Fig. 6-4A), but these are associated with little or no loss of joint space. They are known as *syndesmophytes*, and they occur mainly on the right side of the thoracic spine (possibly because of the pulsating aorta on the left) and on both sides of the lumbar spine. In the cervical spine, syndesmophytes form bridges over the anterior part of the disc spaces. A typical radiographic feature of Forrestier's disease is of "whiskering" at any point where there is a muscle, ligament, or tendinous attachment, and this is often best seen in the pelvis (Fig. 6-4B).

CHARCOT'S JOINTS. The term *neurotrophic joint* implies that the joint has lost pain sensation and proprioception so that the patient can move the joint into abnormal positions because it is pain-free. Charcot described neuropathic joints in patients with tertiary syphilis in 1868 but by far the most common cause of Charcot's joints today is diabetes (see Chap. 9) where the most commonly involved joints are in the feet and ankles (Fig. 6-5). Classically, syringomyelia is associated with neuropathic elbows, whereas tabes dorsalis is associated with Charcot's joints in the spine, knees, and ankles. The radiographic appearance of a neurotrophic joint is unique in that there is marked destruction and disorganization of the joint with all of the classic features of degenerative arthritis exaggerated: but infractions, fractures, subluxations, and dislocations may also occur. This is in the face of marked sclerosis and new bone formation; multiple loose bodies and bone dust may be seen floating within the joint capsule. The only other entity that destroys joints so completely is septic arthritis (see Chap. 4), but this is always associated with marked juxta-articular bone resorption and osteopenia rather than with the obvious new bone formation which is seen in Charcot's joints.

HEMOPHILIA. Another exaggerated form of degenerative arthritis is seen in patients with hemophilia who have recurrent bleeding into one or more joints. The clinical history should provide the diagnosis, but the diagnosis of hemophilic arthritis may be made on radiographic grounds alone. There is obvious joint space narrowing, marked sclerosis, and irregularity of the underlying bone occurring in a young male patient usually with one or two large joints involved asymmetrically. An irregular trabecular pattern may be seen and widening of the epiphysis and metaphysis occurs due to bleeding into the region of the physeal plate as the patient grows from being a child into an adolescent. In the knee, all these changes are associated with widening of the intercondylar notch due to synovial hypertrophy (Fig. 6-6) and in the ankle the characteristic change is an abnormal angulation (tibiotalar tilt) which is due to repeated bleeding into that joint.

HEMOCHROMATOSIS. It is important to remember that deposition of any foreign material, such as a heavy metal or calcification or altered blood into the well-organized crystalline structures of the hyaline cartilage will lead to premature degenerative arthritis. In hemochromatosis, the breakdown products of hemoglobin get deposited all over the body as well as into cartilage where it produces chondrocalcinosis (Table 6-4). The deposition of hemochromatin, however, is also associated with a curious patchy form of hypertrophic osteoarthritis often associated with "squaring off" of the involved bones (Fig. 6-7) which is characteristic of the arthritis seen in hemochromatosis. As a general rule, if one sees changes of osteoarthritis in an unusual joint, one should think of hemochromatosis.

Table 6-4

Chondrocalcinosis
OA
CPPD
Pseudogout
Gout
Hemochromatosis
Hyperparathyroidism (primary & secondary)
Ochronosis
Wilson's disease
Acromegaly
Hypophosphatasia

RHEUMATOID ARTHRITIS AND ITS VARIANTS

The group of rheumatoid diseases is a complex one, and there is considerable overlap between the various conditions. For instance, many patients with psoriatic arthritis go on to develop a more classic form of rheumatoid arthritis and some patients with Reiter's syndrome go on to develop frank ankylosing spondylitis. It is still useful, however, to subdivide the group into "classic" rheumatoid arthritis, psoriatic arthritis, juvenile rheumatoid arthritis, Reiter's syndrome, ankylosing spondylitis, and enteropathic arthritis. Jaccoud's arthritis and the arthritis seen in association with the collagen diseases will also be discussed briefly.

Rheumatoid Arthritis (RA)

Classically rheumatoid arthritis occurs in females aged 20 to 40, but it may begin at any age and the sex ratio is three females to one male. In men, RA may be asymmetrical and not associated with juxta-articular osteopenia, and in blacks (in whom rheumatoid arthritis is rare) it frequently appears to be almost a different disease. Clinically, the patient will first complain of pain, swelling, and early morning stiffness of the hands. This symptomatology often precedes the first radiographic evidence of erosions by several years. The rheumatoid factor is positive in the majority of patients with pure rheumatoid arthritis whereas it is positive in under 6 percent of the normal population. On the other hand, the HLA B27 is positive in less than 10 percent of patients with RA.

The joints involved are classically the small joints of the hands and wrists, feet, and tarsus, but rheumatoid arthritis may involve any joint in the body. It is usually bilateral and symmetrical except in blacks where it may be unilateral, and in some men where it may be bilateral but not symmetrical. Radiographically, soft tissue swelling is apparent particularly around the metacarpophalangeal joints, the wrists, and some proximal interphalangeal joints. The first really positive radiographic finding in rheumatoid arthritis is the presence of juxta-articular erosions, and although these may occur almost anywhere in the hands and feet, often the first erosion to become apparent is on the ulna aspect of the proximal phalanx of the fourth finger at the metacarpophalangeal joint (Fig. 6-8A,B). This erosion can be better seen using either industrial or mammographic film or by using a magnification technique. Early erosions may be seen at other sites such as the ulna styloid or the metatarsophalangeal joints. The erosions of rheumatoid arthritis are difficult to see because they represent actual erosion by the inflamed hypertrophied synovium into the bone, and thus they have poorly defined margins. Often oblique views of the metacarpophalangeal joints ("Brewerton" view or "ballcatcher" view) are necessary to delineate the full extent of the erosions.

Once the disease has become more advanced, joint effusions occur and destruction of the cartilage by pannus formation with subsequent narrowing of the joint cartilage space and juxta-articular osteopenia become apparent (Fig. 6-8C). As the disease progresses, total destruction of many joint spaces and actual disappearance of bone occurs, including marked loss of the ulna styloid (Fig. 6-8D). Ligamentous and soft tissue changes also occur often leading to ulnar deviation of the fingers with "boutonniere" and "swan neck" deformities. These appearances can also occur in the rheumatoid variants although the "seagull" appearance and "cup and pencil" deformities are more common in such conditions as psoriatic arthritis (Fig. 6-9). Since rheumatoid arthritis is an autoimmune disease with overgrowth of synovium and pannus formation occurring throughout the body, any joint or bursa may be affected and the larger weight-bearing joints such as the hips and knees have a characteristic appearance with a combination of erosive rheumatoid changes and sclerotic hypertrophic degenerative changes (Fig. 6-10).

Since any synovial joint or synovially lined bursa may be involved in rheumatoid disease, erosions can be seen at the insertion of the Achilles tendon into the calcaneum, in the sacroiliac joints, symphysis pubis, and apophyseal joints of the spine as well as in the atlantoaxial joint (Fig. 6-11), a particularly important location. The integrity of the articulation of the odontoid process (C2) with the anterior arch of the atlas (C1) depends on the transverse ligament, which has a synovial bursa between it and the posterior surface of the odontoid. Some 45 percent of patients with severe rheumatoid arthritis have synovial hypertrophy in this bursa which ruptures the ligament thus allowing the odontoid to float freely and to move posteriorly and press on the spinal cord producing long tract signs in some patients. Curiously, many patients with atlantoaxial subluxation due to rheumatoid arthritis have no symptoms, but in those patients who have shooting pains down their legs, it is important to stabilize this joint because of the obvious risk of permanent damage or even death due to backward and upward movement of the odontoid through the foramen magnum thus effectively "pithing" the patient. The surgical fusion is usually achieved by wiring the spinous processes of C1, C2, and C3 together.

Rheumatoid arthritis is a whole body disease and although many patients are now being managed successfully with the judicious use of salicylates, steroids, gold, and even cytotoxic drugs, RA can be a very disabling condition leading to long-term hospitalization and severe osteopenia due both to the inflammatory nature of the disease and to disuse. This is a problem when a total joint replacement in a weight-bearing joint such as the knee is contemplated in a patient with severe rheumatoid arthritis. There is a high incidence of fracture postoperatively, usually at the inferior aspect of the prosthesis. Wrist fusions, wrist implants, and sialastic arthroplasties of the small joints of the fingers are on the whole extremely successful and, in fact, can prolong the useful life of many patients with severe rheumatoid arthritis.

Rheumatoid Variants

JUVENILE RHEUMATOID ARTHRITIS (JRA).   This is a type of rheumatoid arthritis which afflicts children and often begins under the age of 5. It is asymmetrical and involves predominantly the larger joints. Juvenile rheumatoid arthritis may begin with a solitary rapidly swelling knee, for example, before going on to involve other joints. Because of the inflammatory nature of this condition, there is often also overgrowth of the physeal plate, epiphysis, and metaphysis with apparent narrowing of the diaphysis, producing a characteristically gracile appearance to the bones. Erosions occur and although initially they may be difficult to see, JRA is a very destructive disease, leading to marked deformities and fusion of many joints (Fig. 6-12). The rheumatoid factor is positive in less than 10 percent of patients with JRA and the HLA B27 is positive in 40 percent. Ten percent of patients with JRA go on to develop the classic symmetrical form of adult rheumatoid arthritis. Juvenile rheumatoid arthritis may be so destructive that if salicylates, gold, and steroids are not successful, the Food and Drug Administration (FDA) has allowed the use of cytotoxic drugs in an attempt to arrest the condition.

Felty's syndrome refers to JRA associated with splenomegaly and neutropenia. *Still's disease* refers to those patients with JRA who have spiking fevers, rash, polyarthralgias, hepatosplenomegaly, and lymphadenopathy, as well as pleuropericarditis and myocarditis.

PSORIATIC ARTHRITIS.   Psoriasis is very common but psoriatic arthritis is fortunately quite rare. But it is possible to have psoriatic arthritis without visible psoriasis, at least for many years. Psoriatic arthritis is slightly more common in women than in men. The age group is somewhat older than with pure rheumatoid arthritis, and whereas the rheumatoid factor is only positive in less than 10 percent of patients with psoriatic arthritis, the HLA B27 is positive in over 80 percent. Characteristically the joint involvement is more peripheral, eccentric, and patchy than in pure rheumatoid arthritis with possibly one proximal interphalangeal joint, one distal interphalangeal joint, and several metacarpophalangeal joints involved (Fig. 6-13A). Although psoriatic arthritis is very destructive, juxta-articular or generalized osteopenia is rare. *Seagulls* are characteristically seen (Fig. 6-9), and this appearance is produced by rapid pannus formation infiltrating between the articular cartilage and the subchondral bone which erodes the bone more centrally than is usually seen in the more slowly growing marginal pannus of classic rheumatoid arthritis. The most characteristic deformity seen in psoriatic arthritis is the *cup and pencil* deformity (Fig. 6-9), which is caused by central erosions of one side of the joint and peripheral erosions on the other side (Fig. 6-13B). Patients with psoriatic arthritis may get involvement of joints other than those in the periphery, and sacroiliitis with syndesmophyte formation as well as apophyseal joint erosions are not uncommonly seen in the spine of patients with psoriatic arthritis. These changes are similar to those seen in enteropathic arthritis.

Another similarity between psoriatic arthritis and enteropathic arthritis (as well as Reiter's syndrome involving the peripheral joints) is the presence of hypertrophic changes. A periosteal reaction may also occur in these three conditions but is particularly common in psoriatic arthritis. Once again, because of the destructiveness of psoriatic arthritis, this is one of the few types of arthritis the FDA has permitted the use of cytotoxic drugs, particularly methotrexate.

THE ARTHRITIS SEEN IN THE COLLAGEN DISEASES SUCH AS LUPUS AND SCLERODERMA.   In the collagen diseases, a vasculitis produces loss of the soft tissues of the tips of the fingers. In scleroderma, amorphous clumps of soft tissue calcification can also be seen. Erosions may be seen, however, at the proximal interphalangeal and metacarpophalangeal joints in many of these patients, and although not symmetrical, the appearance resembles that of early rheumatoid arthritis. In more advanced cases, "seagulls" may also be seen, and this suggests a rheumatoid variant rather than classic rheumatoid arthritis.

JACCOUD'S ARTHRITIS.   This is a rare form of arthritis involving mainly the synovium of the tendons and ligaments. Jaccoud's arthritis occurs in two situations: in association with rheumatic fever and in some patients with lupus erythematosus. The classic finding is marked ulna deviation of the fingers without any other radiographic features of note. In particular, erosions are rarely seen.

ANKYLOSING SPONDYLITIS (AS).   This is a condition which afflicts predominantly young men before the age of 20. Although rare in females in Europe and the east coast of America, about 20 percent of cases of ankylosing spondylitis in California are female. Clinically, ankylosing spondylitis presents with low backache and even at this early stage, the chest expansion is decreased markedly because of the early involvement of the costovertebral joints.
    Radiographically, the first changes occur in the sacroiliac joints (Table 6-5) with irregularity and erosions of both sides, as well as some sclerosis on the iliac side (Fig. 6-14A). Ultimately bony bridging occurs with total fusion of the sacroiliac joints (Fig. 6-14B). The other characteristic changes occur in the spine where the earliest sign of ankylosing spondylitis is squaring off anteriorly of the vertebral bodies due to an active inflammatory process causing bone resorption under the anterior spinal ligament (Fig. 6-15A). Vertebral body osteopenia, ossification of the outermost layer of the annulus fibrosis (Sharpey's fibers), and calcification of many of the spinal ligaments occur inexorably until the spine is straight ("poker spine") and once the intervertebral discs calcify then this is known as a "bamboo spine" (Fig. 6-15B). Moreover, while this process is occurring, the apophyseal and costovertebral joints become involved with erosions and ultimately fuse. Of the patients with ankylosing spondylitis, 100 percent are HLA B27 positive, whereas only 10 percent are rheumatoid factor positive; and 20 percent develop peripheral joint involvement which can resemble an asymmetrical form of rheumatoid arthritis. Another clinical feature of ankylosing spondylitis may be pain and tenderness at the insertion of the Achilles tendon into the os calcis. Synovial overgrowth at this site leads to erosions which are clearly visible on a lateral radiograph of the heel. Calcaneal erosions are also seen in rheumatoid arthritis and Reiter's syndrome (Fig. 6-16), which demonstrates the overlap that is present between all of these conditions.

Table 6-5

Sacroiliac Involvement

Bilateral	Unilateral
Symmetrical	
AS	Gout
Reiter's syndrome	Infections, tuberculosis, pyogenic
Enteropathic	OA
Asymmetrical	
JRA	
Psoriatic	
RA	

The complications of ankylosing spondylitis include fractures of the spine (due to the severe osteopenia), recurrent chest infections (due to poor respiratory motion secondary to the fusion of the costovertebral joints), and the rare occurrence of aortic regurgitation (due to rheumatoid nodules laid down in the aortic valve ring). The old treatment for AS was radiotherapy to the thoracolumbar region which halted the progression of the disease, but produced an increased incidence of leukemia in the recipients. Modern forms of therapy include the use of salicylates and other antiinflammatory agents and back bracing and exercises in order to allow the spine to fuse upright.

REITER'S SYNDROME.   This condition is named after a Prussian army physician whose regiment was infected with dysentery in 1915. One soldier developed urethritis, uveitis, and back pain. Some years later, after several other similar cases had been described, Reiter's name was attached to the triad of sacroiliitis, uveitis, and urethritis. The sacroiliitis resembles that seen in ankylosing spondylitis with erosions and irregularity of the sacroiliac joints bilaterally and symmetrically, although the iliac sclerosis is more marked in both Reiter's syndrome and enteropathic arthritis than in pure AS (Fig. 6-17). Patients with Reiter's syndrome are virtually always male, usually aged between 15 and 35, are rheumatoid factor negative and HLA B27 positive (90 percent of cases). Although the majority of patients recover spontaneously, some may go on to fusion of the sacroiliac joints and 10 percent develop peripheral joint involvement similar to rheumatoid arthritis. A further 10 percent go on to develop spinal fusion and changes similar to true ankylosing spondylitis. Erosions around the calcaneum are not uncommon (Fig. 6-16).

ENTEROPATHIC ARTHRITIS.   About 10 percent of patients with either ulcerative colitis or regional enteritis will develop the signs and symptoms of sacroiliitis, or spinal arthritis equivalent to ankylosing spondylitis, or have peripheral joint changes similar to those seen in any of the rheumatoid variants (with "seagulling" of the small joints of the fingers). The classic changes occur in the spine where syndesmophytes are common, and in the sacroiliac joints where there are erosions, irregularity, and iliac sclerosis (Fig. 6-18). Patients with enteropathic arthritis are rheumatoid factor negative and 75 percent are HLA B27 positive.

Final Comment on Rheumatoid Arthritis and the Rheumatoid Variants

There is a large degree of overlap between pure rheumatoid arthritis and its variants. Although it may seem rather pedantic to separate all these conditions from each other, it is in fact important because the prognosis of such diseases as rheumatoid arthritis and psoriatic arthritis, Reiter's syndrome, and ankylosing spondylitis are totally different. So when faced with a patient who has "arthritis," take an adequate clinical history, do the rheumatoid factor and HLA B27, and look carefully at the x-rays. As a final radiologic comment, there is probably no such thing as a good "arthritis survey" but it is important to x-ray painful joints using high resolution films or a magnification technique if an extremity is involved.

GOUT

Gout occurs as a result of a breakdown in the purine metabolism, allowing the serum uric acid to rise. Eventually it will reach the stage of supersaturation in the bloodstream with sodium monohydrate monourate crystals deposited all over the body. Secondary gout occurs as a result of a number of metabolic disasters, including leukemia and the use of cytotoxic drugs in cancer patients, for example, where excessive tissue breakdown leads to a rise in serum uric acid and eventually to gout if this situation persists. If the deposition of urate crystals occurs in the soft tissues, there is an intense inflammatory reaction, marked erythema, soft tissue swelling, and severe pain. Ultimately soft tissue calcification occurs, and this is then known as a "tophus" (from the Greek word "toph" or "tufa" meaning a calcarious limestone deposit). If the urate crystals get deposited in the synovium, then gouty arthritis ensues. Typically, an overweight, wine-drinking, middle-aged male such as Samuel Pepys or Henry VIII could and did develop gout, but, in fact, there are many thin people who have an inborn error of purine metabolism who also suffer from gout. Gout is ten times more common in men than in women. It occurs from age 30 onwards and involves classically the first metatarsophalangeal joint, but of course may involve any joint in the body.

The typical radiographic features of gout are a destructive form of arthritis with large erosions which can be centrally or peripherally placed (Fig. 6-19A). The classic radiograph hallmark of gout is a cyst which is away from the joint (Fig. 6-19B), and this, of course, cannot occur in rheumatoid arthritis (which is a synovial disease) or in osteoarthritis (where the cysts are subchrondral and contain synovial fluid). These erosions are associated with marked new bone formation and sclerosis and thus have well-defined margins, unlike the erosions seen in RA. Effusions and chondrocalcinosis (Table 6-4) also occur (Fig. 6-19C).

PSEUDOGOUT

Pseudogout is a condition of older people and clinically resembles gout, hence the name. The sex incidence is equal and pseudogout is more common in patients over 40. It is bilateral and often symmetrical and involves primarily the larger joints. Clinically the patient will complain of pain and swelling in the knees, elbows, or wrists and on examination there is marked soft tissue swelling with erythema.

Radiologically, the hallmark of pseudogout is chondrocalcinosis (Fig. 6-20). In the older textbooks of radiology, the two terms were used synonymously (Table 6-4). The cartilage calcification is related to the presence of calcium pyrophosphate crystals in the joint, but this substance is also found in most cases of degenerating cartilage such as is seen in osteoarthritis and should not be considered a specific finding for pseudogout.

CALCIUM PYROPHOSPHATE DISEASE (CPPD)

This condition has been described recently as being a separate entity from both degenerative arthritis and pseudogout. It probably represents, however, a specific form of osteoarthritis in which chondrocalcinosis occurs due to the deposition of calcium pyrophosphate crystals.

FINAL COMMENT

The vast majority of patients who present with "arthritis" have a type of arthritis that is clinically diagnosable. The radiographs help to confirm this diagnosis as well as to demonstrate the degree of damage and distortion of the joints involved. Of the remaining patients, a careful consideration of the radiographic features as well as taking into account the biochemical findings should reveal the correct diagnosis (Table 6-6).

Table 6-6

An Approach to Arthritis

	OA	RA	Gout	Pseudogout
Age of onset (yrs.)	50+	20–40	40+	40+
Sex	♀ = ♂	♀ 3:1 ♂	♂ 10:1 ♀	♂ 3:1 ♀
Clinical	Painful deformities	Early morning stiffness: symmetry	Acute attacks: sodium urate xtals:tophi	Acute attacks: sodium pyrophosphate crystals
Rheumatoid factor	–	+	–	–
HLA-B-27	–	–	–	–
Location	Big joints hips/ knees/ shoulders	Small joints MCP/PIP	Various: 1st MTP	Big joints knees/ ankles/ wrists/ disc spaces
Symmetry	Fairly	Yes	No	Usually
Initial radiographs	↓ joint space squaring off	S.T. swelling and ↑ joint space	S.T. swelling with or without calcification	Joint effusions
Joint space later	↓ and osteophytes	↓	↓	↕
Calcification	No	No	Soft tissue: tophi	Chondrocalcinosis
Osteoporosis	No	Juxta-articular → generalized	No	No
Cysts & Erosions	Central cysts	Peripheral: at edges of joint	Punched out with sclerotic margins	None
Other features	Osteophytes, sclerosis Heberden's nodes loss of joint space, loose bodies	Ulnar deviation, destruction subluxations and telescoping fingers, bony anklylosis, A/A, subluxation, large joints, knees and hips	Large cysts may be away from joint: disorganized joints, tophi in earlobes and elbows	Usually no other signs. May have fever and look septic

Also note: UC: 18%, SI joint changes → RA, 4% → AS. Crohn's Disease: 5% → RA.

An Approach to Arthritis (Cont.)

Psoriatic	Ankylosis Spondylitis	Reiters Syndrome	Juvenile RA
30+	20–30	15–30	Under 5
♀ > ♂	♂ 10:1 ♀	98% ♂	♂ = ♀
Chronic: associated with psoriasis	Pain over sacroiliac joints → back → neck	Urethritis, uveitis, and arthritis	Severe pain and deformity, fever rash
−	−	−	−
+ 30%	+ 90–100%	+ 80%	−
Various: DIP and PIP	SI joints → spine → heels	SI joints → heels toes and large joints	Large joints and wrists
No	Yes	No	No
S.T. swelling and ↑ joint space	Widening and sclerosis of sacroiliac space	−	S.T. swelling and effusions
↓	Fusion of SI joints, costovertebral and apophyseal joints	Erosion of SI joints	↑ → ↓ ankylosis
Calcification in spinal ligaments in 10%	Spinal ligaments	No	No
No	In vertebral bodies	May be regional	Generalized (severe)
≡ RA	Not visible	Calcaneal spur/SI joints	Peripheral ≡ RA severe
Mutilation: pencil and cup deformities 60% → RA and few → AS large joints spine & SI joints	AR kyphosis respiratory problems → RA 20%	May → RA or → AS	60% burn out; 30% bony ankylosis; 25% subacute; →10% RA; →4% AS

REFERENCES

Arnett FC Jr: The implications of HL-A W27, an editorial. Ann Intern Med 84:94–95, 1976

Forrester DM, Brown JC, Nesson JW: The Radiology of Joint Disease, 2nd ed. Philadelphia, Saunders, 1978

Griffiths HJ, Gobien RP: A logical approach to arthritis. Aust J Radiol 22:60–69, 1978

Resnick D: Rheumatoid arthritis of the wrist. Med. Radiogr Photogr 52:50–88, 1976

The Arthritis Foundation: Primer on Rheumatoid Diseases. New York, 1964

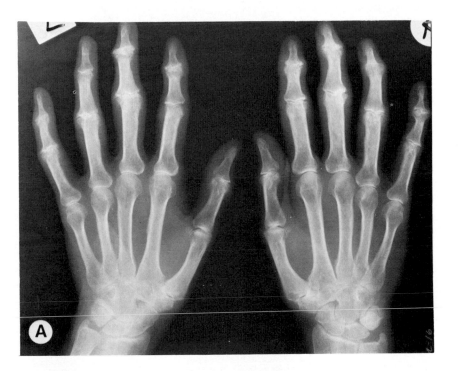

Heberdeen's
nodes
Bouchard's

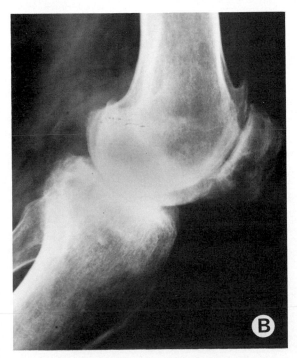

FIGURE 6-1. *Osteoarthritis.* **A.** Hands. There is narrowing, sclerosis, and osteophyte formation at many of the distal interphalangeal (DIP) joints. Similar but less severe changes are present in the proximal interphalangeal (PIP) joints and at the first carpometacarpal (CMP) joint bilaterally. **B.** Knee. Note the joint space narrowing, sclerosis, and osteophyte formation in all three compartments of the knee, particularly involving the patellofemoral joint.

FIGURE 6-2. *Osteoarthritis: Geodes.*   There are large subchondral cysts (arrows) on either side of the narrowed sclerotic hip joint in this 70-year-old man. Note the "ring" of osteophytes around the femoral head (curved arrows).

Osteophytes:

1 Periosteal

2 Capsular
collar sign

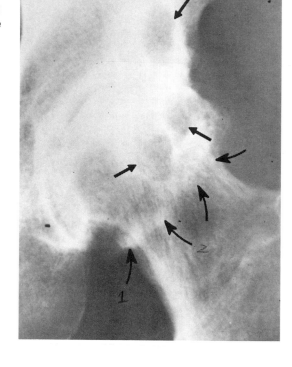

FIGURE 6-3. *Secondary Osteoarthritis.*   This 42-year-old woman suffered from a slipped capital femoral epiphysis at the age of 12 and now has developed secondary osteoarthritis with large osteophytes, sclerosis, and joint space narrowing in her left hip. Note the obvious deformity of the femoral head and neck with the head "slipped" medially (arrow). The right hip is normal.

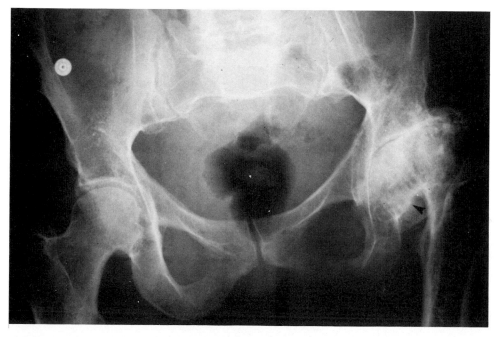

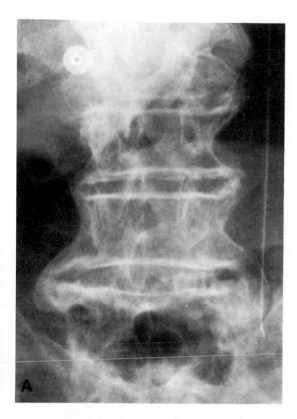

FIGURE 6-4. *Forrestier's Disease (DISH).* **A.**
Spine. There are large bridging syndesmophytes
surrounding many of the lower lumbar disc spaces
which are noted to be normal in width. This is
characteristic of DISH. **B.** Pelvis. There is marked
"whiskering" at every point where muscles, tendons, or ligaments are inserted into this 55-year-
old man's pelvis. Note the hypertrophic changes
over the roof of both acetabuli in association with
normal joint spaces in the hips as well as the ossification in one of the saroiliac ligaments.

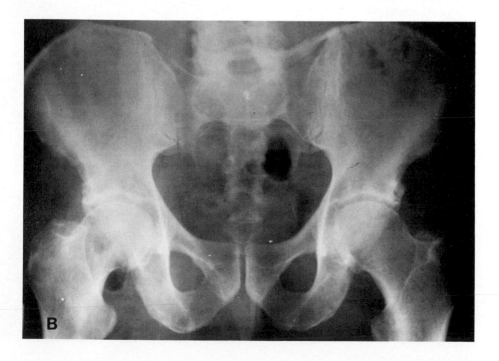

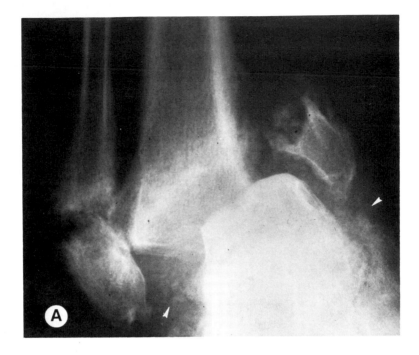

FIGURE 6-5. *Charcot's Joints.*   **A.** Ankle. Note the total disorganization of this ankle joint with obvious destruction of the distal tibia, fractures of both malleoli and an extreme angulation to the tibiotalar joint. This is all seen in association with increased bone sclerosis and plentiful bone dust and free-floating fragments in the distended joint capsule (arrows). This patient had tabes dorsalis. **B.** Spine. This 48-year-old female also had tabes dorsalis and has extreme disorganization of the lower lumbar spine with apparent disintegration of the body of L4. There is marked sclerosis and bits of bone are apparently floating all around the spine thus producing a "tumbled bricks" appearance typical of a Charcot spine.

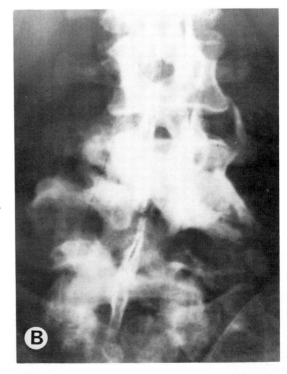

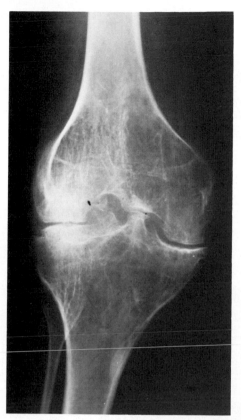

FIGURE 6-6. *Hemophilia: Knee.* This 27-year-old male with severe hemophilia has involvment of both knees, one hip, and one elbow. This knee shows the characteristic appearance—thin "gracile" diaphysis, widened metaphysis, and epiphysis with a coarse disorganized trabecular pattern. The joint is narrowed and irregular with widening and destruction of the intercondylar notch. Note the synovial erosions of the edge of both the femur and the tibia.

FIGURE 6-7. *Hemochromatosis: Hand.* There is evidence of osteoarthritis in the second and third metacarpophalangeal joints bilaterally in association with squaring off and beaking of the metacarpal heads. The hands are otherwise normal for a patient of 53 apart from some early degenerative changes seen in a number of interphalangeal joints. This is a characteristic appearance of hemochromatosis involving the hands. Note that this patient does not have chondrocalcinosis.

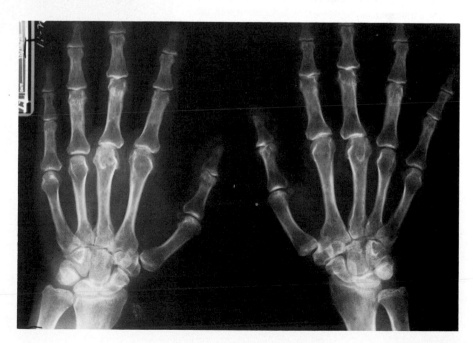

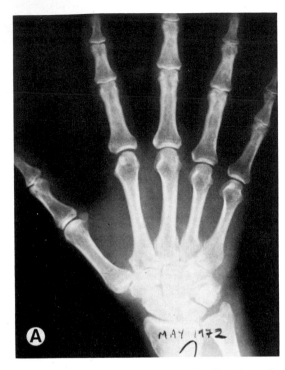

FIGURE 6-8. *Rheumatoid Arthritis: Hands.* **A.**
Very early changes in a female patient of 32 (film
date 10/5/72). Note the very discrete erosions at
many of the metacarpophalangeal joints as well as
the soft-tissue swelling around these joints and
wrist.

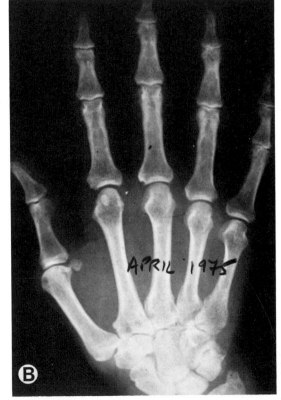

FIGURE 6-8B. The same patient in April 1975.
The erosions are now more obvious and better
defined, and there is some juxta-articular osteoporosis. (For Figs. 6-8C,D see facing page.)

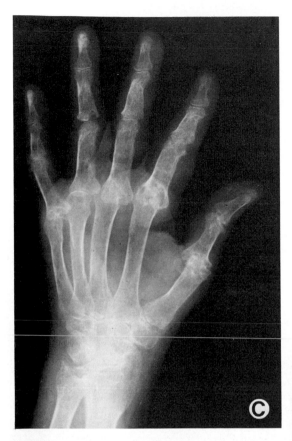

FIGURE 6-8C. More severe rheumatoid arthritis in a different patient. Note the markedly destructive nature of this condition with loss of joint space, erosive destruction of many of the carpal bones and erosions at many synovial insertions. This 50-year-old woman has subluxation of many of the metacarpophalangeal joints as well as widespread osteopenia.

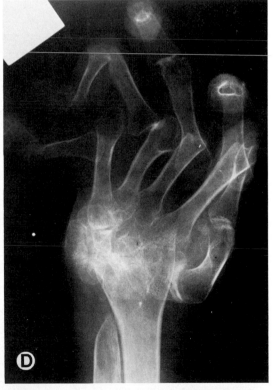

FIGURE 6-8D. Severe rheumatoid arthritis. This 63-year-old female has total disorganization of the carpus, loss of the ulna styloid, and dislocation of the metacarpophalangeal joint. Note the severe osteoporosis.

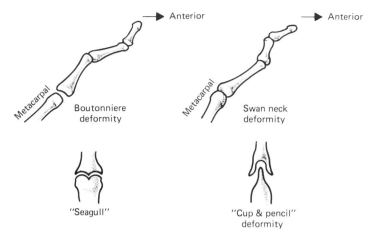

FIGURE 6-9.   Illustrations of boutonniere and swan neck deformities, seagulls, and cup and pencil deformities.

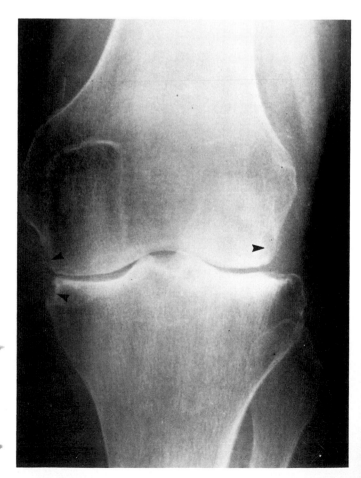

FIGURE 6-10. *Rheumatoid Arthritis: Knee.*   There is symmetrical narrowing of both medial and lateral compartments in the knees of this 48-year-old woman with rheumatoid arthritis. Note the marginal tibial erosion as well as erosions of the distal femoral condyles (arrows) and the lack of sclerosis and osteophyte formation.

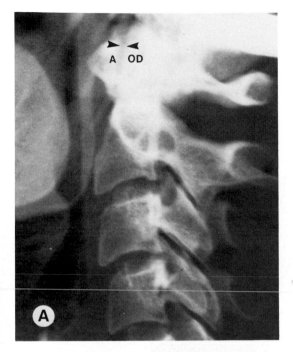

FIGURE 6-11. *Rheumatoid Arthritis: Atlantoaxial Joint.* **A.** Normal for comparison. Note the close approximation of the front of the odontoid (OD) to the back of the arch of the atlas (A). This space should be no greater than 2mm. **B.** This 43-year-old man with severe rheumatoid arthritis has atlantoaxial separation. Note on this tomogram the OD is not only shifted posteriorly but is eroded (curved arrows). There is a 9-mm separation of this atlantoaxial joint which is a characteristic finding in severe rheumatoid arthritis.

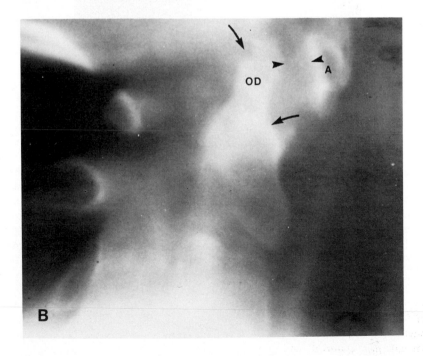

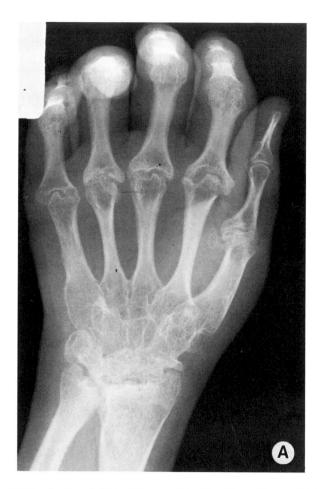

FIGURE 6-12. *JRA.*   **A.** Hand: This 17-year-old girl with a 12-year history of JRA has fusion of the carpus and deformities of most of the other joints, including flexion contractures of the fingers. Note the gracile nature of the long bones. **B.** Elbow: There is marked destruction of the left elbow joint in the same patient with large erosions of the humeral condyles and the proximal ulna and apparent loss of the radial head. Again note the thin diaphyses. **C.** Pelvis (same patient). There is fusion of both hip joints with distortion of the upper femurs. The left sacroiliac joint is also eroded and narrowed. (See facing page for Figs. 6-12B, C.)

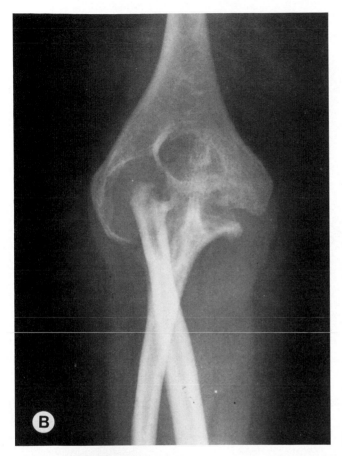

FIGURE 6-12, continued.

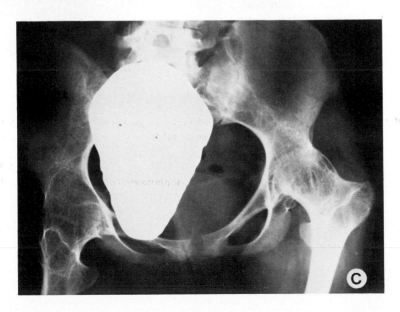

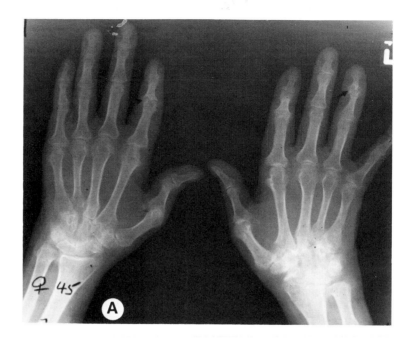

FIGURE 6-13. *Psoriatic Arthritis.*   **A.** Hands. This woman of 45 has had psoriasis for 20 years but only developed arthritis 2 years previously. Note the patchy asymmetrical involvement with seagulls (arrows) and marked loss of joint cartilage space in one wrist. **B.** Feet. Cup and pencil deformities can be seen in many of the interphalangeal joints of the toes in this 61-year-old man with a 10-year history of psoriatic arthritis. Note how destructive this form of arthritis can be.

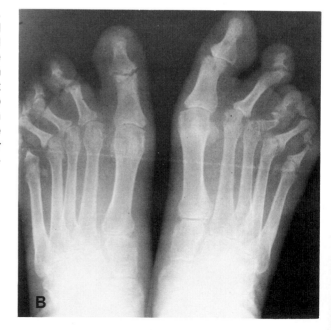

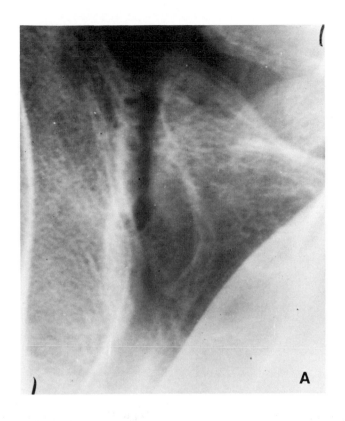

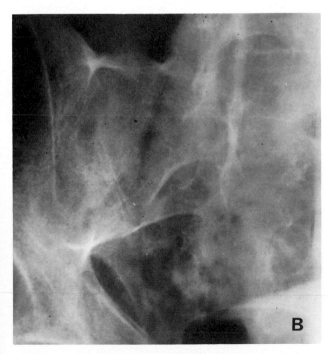

FIGURE 6-14. *Ankylosing Spondylitis: Sacroiliac Joints.* **A.** Early. This 21-year-old man had complained of low backache for 3 years. This oblique view shows marked irregularity of the sacroiliac joint with horizontal new bone formation as a prelude to bridging. Notice that there is relatively little sclerosis. **B.** Late. This sacroiliac joint is completely fused in this 56-year-old man with a 30-year history of ankylosing spondylitis. Note the calcifications and ossifications in the spinal ligaments.

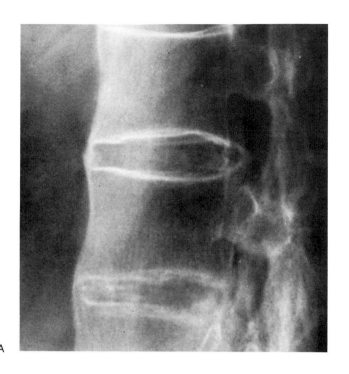

A

FIGURE 6-15. *Ankylosing Spondylitis: Spine.* **A.** Early. There is squaring off of the anterior end plate, ossification in the anterior spinal ligament and relative osteopenia in the vertebral bodies of this young male patient. There is also some disc calcification. **B.** Late. Bamboo Spine. The spine is straight and severely osteopenic with calcification in the discs and ossification in the ligaments. This is the same patient as illustrated in Figure 6-14B.

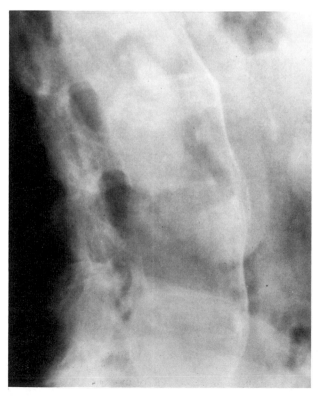

B

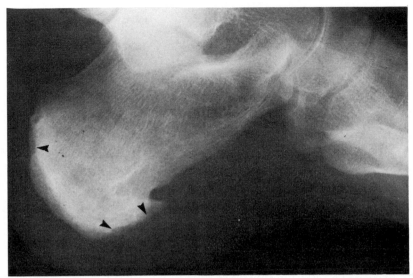

enthesopathy

FIGURE 6-16. *Reiter's Syndrome: Erosion of Os Calcis.* Erosions of the heel (arrows) can be seen in ankylosing spondylitis, rheumatoid arthritis, and in Reiter's syndrome. The erosions may occur either at the insertion of the Achilles tendon or at the origin of the plantar fascia.

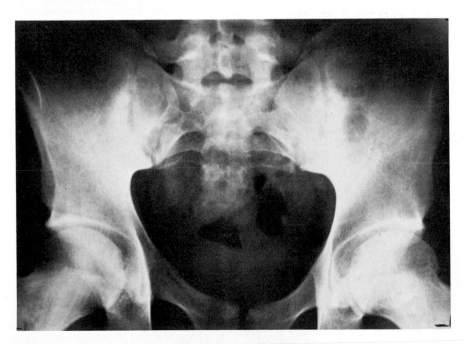

FIGURE 6-17. *Reiter's Syndrome: Sacroiliitis.* This 24-year-old man presented with low back pain and uveitis. Both sacroiliac joints show evidence of erosions with marked sclerosis on the iliac side of the joint.

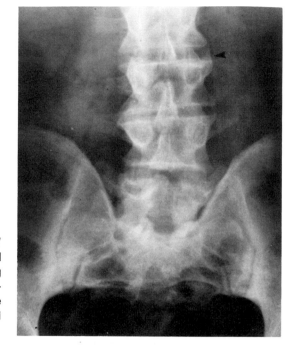

FIGURE 6-18. *Enteropathic Arthritis: Spine and Sacroiliac Joints.*   There is narrowing and sclerosis in association with erosions involving both sacroiliac joints. A large syndesmophyte (arrow) and several smaller ones may be seen in the lumbar spine. This 29-year-old man had suffered from ulcerative colitis for 5 years.

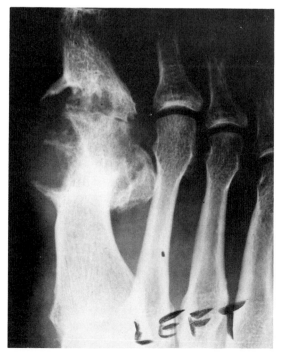

FIGURE 6-19. *Gout.*   **A,B.** The feet of a 58-year-old man who enjoyed drinking wine. The left foot (A) shows the characteristic changes of gout involving the first metatarsophalangeal joint with erosions and destructive changes as well as well-marked spiky hypertrophic changes. (For Figs. 6-19B,C see facing page.)

A

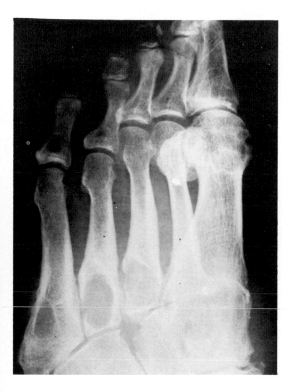

FIGURE 6-19B. The right foot shows large centrally placed, well marginated lucencies on the proximal metatarsals away from the joints as well as more characteristic changes of gout elsewhere.

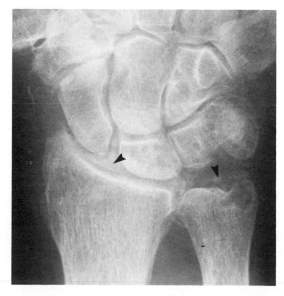

FIGURE 6-19C. Wrist. There are erosions and cysts in many of the carpal bones as well as in the ulna styloid in this 78-year-old patient with long-standing gout. Note the chondrocalcinosis (arrows).

C

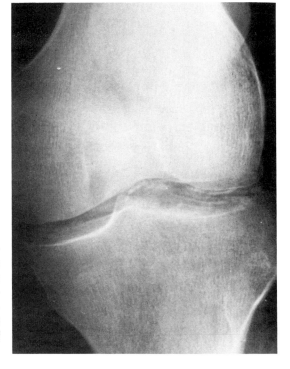

FIGURE 6-20. *Pseudogout: Knees.* This 72-year-old man has marked chondrocalcinosis in many joints in his body. His knees show both hyaline cartilage and meniscal calcification. Clinically, he presented with symmetrical pain, swelling, and erythema. Radiographically, he has chondrocalcinosis and hence the diagnosis of pseudogout.

SEVEN

Bone Tumors

Primary bone tumors are quite rare, and in an introductory text it is probably irrelevant to provide detailed descriptions of each of them. For the sake of completeness, however, brief *outlines* of the more common benign and malignant bone tumors are given, followed by a discussion of tumors of the hematopoietic system and finally metastases. For those interested in pursuing the subject of bone tumors further, one of the best authorities is published by the Armed Forces Institute of Pathology (AFIP).

When faced with a radiograph of a bone tumor, it is necessary to decide first if the tumor is benign or malignant. In order to accomplish this, it is important to elicit any relevant clinical information and then to assess the radiographic appearance with great care. The age of the patient is important (Table 7-1) because certain tumors occur at certain ages. For instance, Ewing's sarcoma is rare after 20 and metastases rare before 40. The sex of the patient is not particularly relevant, although for instance, osteoid osteoma and osteogenic sarcoma are more common in males, whereas aneurysmal bone cysts and giant cell tumors are more common in females. It is important to know if there is any pain associated with the lesion, for if there is, there is a higher probability of the tumor being malignant. Malignant tumors are also associated with soft tissue swelling and masses as well as systemic signs and symptoms. For example, an elevated ESR frequently occurs in Ewing's sarcoma. If the lesion is thought to be a metastasis, certain primary tumors only occur in certain sexes, such as uterus and cervix in women and prostate in men. Some tumors are far more common in one sex than the other, such as breast in women and lung in men (Table 7-2).

Table 7-1

Typical Age Range of the
Occurance of Bone Tumors

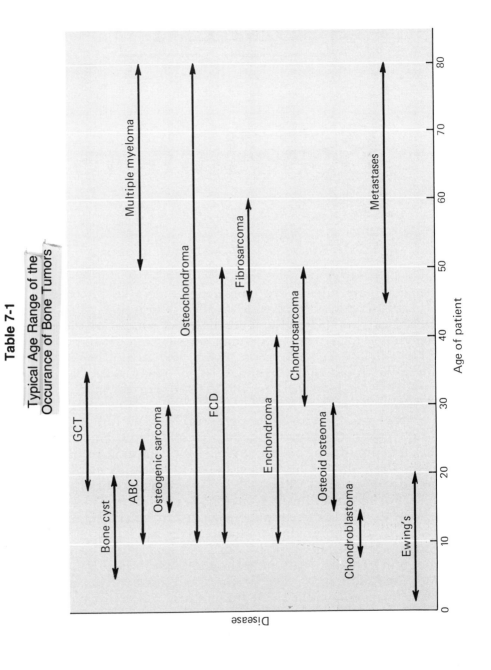

Table 7-2

Metastases		
	Male	*Female*
Lytic	Lung	Breast
	Kidney	Lung
	Bladder	Kidney
	Colon	Uterus/Cervix
Blastic	Prostate	Breast
	Breast	
	Glioma	
Mixed	Lung	Breast
		Uterus/Cervix

Solitary expansatile	*Peripheral*
Kidney	Lung
Thyroid	
Lung	

The radiograph must be scrutinized with great care and certain features should be noted and help should be sought also from the clinical and biochemical data. Radiographic surveys and radioisotopic bone scans should be obtained where relevant. Look to see if the lesion is solitary (benign or malignant) or multiple (usually malignant). Note which bone is involved and if it is a flat bone (more likely to be cartilaginous in origin) or long bone (more likely to be osseous or fibrous tissue in origin). See which part of the bone is involved (Table 7-3); see whether the lesion is epiphyseal (chondroblastoma), epiphyseal and metaphyseal (giant cell tumor), metaphyseal (most tumors) or diaphyseal. The only primary diaphyseal tumors are the round cell or plasma cell tumors, although metastases are usually diaphyseal and some benign tumors "migrate" from the metaphysis into the diaphysis, for example, unicameral bone cysts and enchondromas. Look at the lesion carefully. See if there is evidence of true soft tissue swelling or not, but this must be differentiated from soft tissue displacement which occurs in benign tumors. Decide if the lesion is central (unicameral bone cyst) or eccentric (aneurysmal bone cyst or giant cell tumor) and see if the lesion expands the bone. If it does check to see if the cortex is intact (benign) or eroded and destroyed (malignant). Define the margins of the lesion. Look to see if the lesion has a well-defined sclerotic margin (benign), a thin eggshell rim with clear-cut margins (benign), or if the lesion has poorly defined margins or no margins at all (malignant).

Table 7-3

Site of the Tumor

Epiphyseal	Chondroblastoma
Physeal (i.e. metaphyseal into epiphysis)	Giant cell tumor
Metaphyseal to diaphyseal	Unicameral bone cyst and enchondroma
Diaphyseal	Round cell tumors (reticulum cell sarcoma, Ewing's sarcoma, multiple myeloma) and metastases
Metaphyseal	Everything else

Look for a periosteal reaction or new bone formation which suggests that the tumor is malignant. This reaction may take three principle forms: (1) an *onionskin* or *laminated* type most often seen in Ewing's sarcoma; (2) a *Codman's triangle* which infers that the tumor is very fast growing and has exploded out of the bone into the soft tissues (osteogenic sarcoma); (3) *new bone formation* within the tumor mass itself, which is also very suggestive of the tumor being malignant. What are the contents of the lesion? A totally lucent tumor infers that it contains myxoid tissue, fibrous tissue, uncalcified cartilage, or unossified osteoid. On the other hand, if it contains dense material, it must be decided if this is *calcification*, which appears denser than bone, is white and flocculent, and seen in cartilaginous tumors both benign and malignant; or *ossification*, which has a more "trabeculated" or lamellar structure that is seen in osseous tumors such as osteogenic sarcoma.

It should be possible from this information to decide if the lesion is benign or malignant (Table 7-4). Thus, a classic benign tumor could be described as being metaphyseal, centrally placed with expansion and scalloping of the cortex, with clear-cut margins and a sharply defined transition zone between the tumor and the underlying normal bone, i.e., a

Table 7-4

Benign vs Malignant

	Benign	Malignant
Size	Small	Large
Soft tissue mass	None	Large
Periosteal reaction	Rare	Common
Margins	Sclerotic	None
Zone of transition	Narrow	Wide
Trabeculation	Yes	No
Cortical destruction	Rare	Usual
Overall appearance	Geographic	Moth-eaten or permeative

unicameral bone cyst. A typical malignant tumor could be metaphyseal, eccentric with a large soft tissue mass containing amorphous irregular ossification or calcification, having burst through and destroyed the cortex, and having a Codman's triangle (osteogenic sarcoma). At this stage of the discussion it is important to remember two facts: (1) *for every primary bone tumor, you will see 20 metastases,* (2) *certain metastases can look benign such as those from hypernephroma and thyroid carcinoma.* Solitary myeloma of bone (plasmacytoma) also often looks benign. But certain benign lesions such as giant cell tumor and villonodular synovitis can appear malignant. If you read this chapter carefully and learn the correct approach to a bone tumor, it is possible to diagnose correctly about 95 percent of all bone tumors. Lodwick, using a computer, has achieved this (see references).

TUMORS OF OSTEOBLASTIC ORIGIN

Osteoid Osteoma

Age: 20–30.

Sex: more common in males.

Site: Metaphysis; bones involved: femur, talus, tibia, patella, *rarely* spine, *never* skull and clavicles.

Symptoms: patient wakes up with pain in the middle of the night relieved by aspirin.

Radiographic appearance: a lucent nidus, often with a surrounding cortical rind (Fig. 7-1), but this depends on whether the tumor is in cortical or cancellous bone.

Treatment: disappears if left alone for 4 to 6 years; salicylates; surgical removal of nidus.

Comments: this is benign and may in fact be an inflammatory process rather than a true neoplasm.

Differential diagnosis: tuberculous abscess, chronic osteomyelitis (Brodie's abscess), or sclerosing osteomyelitis of Garre.

Osteosarcoma

It is important to realize that there are a number of different types of osteosarcoma and that this term covers the classic "osteogenic sarcoma," parosteal osteosarcoma, telangiectatic osteosarcoma, juxtacortical osteosarcoma, and the sarcoma seen in Paget's disease and following irradiation.

Classic "Osteogenic Sarcoma"

Age: 10–25.

Sex: more common in men.

Site: metaphyseal

Bones involved: 75 percent at knee (of which the majority occur in the distal femur).

Symptoms: pain for 3 months following trauma.

Radiographic appearance: very destructive, large soft tissue mass and right-angled spiculation ("sunray") or new bone formation in the mass often with a Codman's triangle (Fig. 7-2A,B).

Treatment: surgical removal with or without chemotherapy, with or without radiotherapy, and with or without immunotherapy.

Prognosis: five-year survival rate ±10 percent, although the more aggressive forms of chemotherapy in carefully chosen patients is apparently associated with a 5-year survival rate better than 80 percent; otherwise metastases go to other bones, lungs and liver.

Comment: often occurs in taller children (and larger dogs) at time of growth spurt.

Variants

1. *Multifocal osteosarcoma:* Children with multiple dense metaphyseal lesions; poor prognosis.
2. *Parosteal osteosarcoma:* Originates in periosteum in somewhat older patients (25–40) and is much rarer than classic osteosarcoma. Seventy percent occur in the metaphysis of the lower femur. Radiographically, it appears as though someone has "poured" dense white bone around the original bone and the diagnosis is confirmed by finding a lucent line in the tumor. This represents the periosteum which is fibrous tissue and hence lucent (Fig. 7-2C). Parosteal osteosarcoma has a 5-year survival rate of 60 to 80 percent and is treated by amputation.
3. *Juxtacortical osteosarcoma:* Rare but originates at the margin of the periosteum and the cortex; very destructive and locally invasive (Fig. 7-2D). Occurs in older patients and is treated with amputation. There is a 50 to 60 percent 5-year survival rate.
4. *Telangiectatic osteosarcoma:* Rare, malignant, and radioresistant; metaphyseal and usually appears lucent and destructive; prognosis very poor.

5. *Sarcoma in Paget's disease:* This is usually not a pure osteosarcoma and is actually extremely rare (Fig. 7-2E); poor prognosis.
6. *Sarcoma following irradiation:* Follows exposure to radium in radium dial painters or chemists; from 10 to 50 years after exposure; also seen postthorium administration or following external radiation for benign tumors, chronic infections, or metastases, 6 to 14 years later; poor prognosis.

TUMORS OF CARTILAGINOUS ORIGIN

There are many benign cartilaginous tumors but only two are common:

Enchondroma

Age: 10–40.

Sex: male more than female.

Site: metaphysis, diaphysis.

Bones involved: 50 percent of enchondromas occur in the small bones of the hands, but they may also be seen in humerus, femur, ribs, and feet.

Radiographic appearance: area of lucency with expansion and thinning of the cortex, and containing flecks of amorphous calcification (Fig. 7-3).

Treatment: curettage, but there is a risk of malignancy many years later, particularly in those enchondromas occurring in long bones.

Osteochondroma (exostosis)

Age: any.

Site: metaphyseal.

Bones involved: long bones, 50 percent at knee and shoulder.

Radiographic appearance: smooth bony outgrowth with either a clear-cut edge or surrounded by flocculent calcification (Fig. 7-4). There are three types (Fig. 7-5A) of which the type with a calcified cartilaginous cap is premalignant.

Treatment: remove if troublesome.

Comment: there is a clever theory to explain the origin of osteochondromas (Fig. 7-5B). Also note that there is a familial type of multiple osteochondromatosis in which there is a high risk of malignancy (chondrosarcoma).

Chondroblastoma

This is the only truly epiphyseal tumor and appears as a lucency in the epiphysis and contains speckled calcifications. These occur in young children before the physeal plate fuses (Fig. 7-6). They are rare.

Chondromyxoid fibroma

These are benign, expansatile, metaphyseal tumors containing cartilage, myxoid, and fibrous tissue. These occur near the knee, in the pelvis, in the metacarpals, and classically in a rib.

Chondrosarcoma

Age: 35–50, or older in patients with a so-called secondary chondrosarcoma.

Sex: males predominate.

Site: metaphyseal in long bones, central in flat bones.

Bones involved: pelvis, ribs, upper femur, and shoulder girdle.

Radiographic appearance: slow growing, large soft-tissue mass with or without flocculent calcifications; destructive to underlying bone; may have dense endosteal or periosteal reaction (Fig. 7-7).

Treatment: removal, radiotherapy.

Prognosis: poor but 10-year survival rate is 35 percent.

Comments: many of these may be secondary to a preexisting "benign" cartilaginous tumor, such as an enchondroma or osteochondroma.

TUMORS OF FIBROUS TISSUE ORIGIN

One of the most common benign bone tumors is a fibrocortical defect, and this has acquired many names depending on its site and its size (such as fibro-osseous bone defect and nonossifying fibroma). The malignant tumor of fibrous tissue origin is the fibrosarcoma.

Fibrocortical defect (FCD)

Age: 10–50, apparently many fill in spontaneously and disappear as the patient ages.

Site: metaphyseal; lower femur, upper and lower tibia.

Radiographic appearance: soap bubble appearance at edge of bone, "splitting" the cortex (Fig. 7-8). They may be small or large, single or multiple and are probably secondary to a disturbance of ossification at the physeal plate. They are benign, common, and of no significance.

Fibrosarcoma

Age: 45–60.

Site: metaphyseal in long bones, flat bones, and soft tissues.

Bones involved: knee, pelvis.

Radiographic appearance: slow-growing, soft-tissue mass with either total destruction or erosion of bone (Fig. 7-9). If the fibrosarcoma originates from the soft tissues, it may "impinge" on a long bone and produce pressure effects.

Treatment: removal.

Prognosis: poor; 10-year survival rate 10 to 15 percent.

TUMORS OF MISCELLANEOUS ORIGIN

Now let us consider four benign-looking cystic lesions of bone.

Hemangioma of bone

This has three classic appearances: (1) if it involves a *vertebral body,* it produces vertical striations; (This is part of the differential diagnosis of an "ivory vertebra" and is common.) (2) if it involves the *skull,* a "sunrise" appearance occurs; and (3) if it involves a *long bone,* it produces a group of soap bubble or honeycomb lesions which may surround a joint. This last appearance is a rare form of hemangiomatosis.

Solitary or unicameral bone cyst

Age: 2–20, but disappear with age

Sex: three times as common in males

Site: metaphysis into diaphysis

Bones involved: upper humerus and upper femur (75 percent of cysts)

Radiographic appearance: central in long bones with thinning of cortex, symmetrical expansion, and clear-cut margins with underlying bone. If the patient presents with a fracture through a unicameral bone cyst, look for a fallen fragment (Fig. 7-10).

Treatment: curette and pack with bone chips, although 30 percent recur, but 15 percent heal after fracturing.

Aneurysmal bone cyst (ABC)

Age: 6–25.

Sex: more common in females.

Sites: metaphyseal in long bones, but also rarely occur in vertebrae and flat bones.

Radiographic appearance: asymmetric with a periosteal "blowout" and "aneurysmal" appearance. Usually unilocular (Fig. 7-11).

Treatment: curettage.

Prognosis: excellent.

Comment: many authorities consider that aneurysmal bone cysts are not primary tumors but occur secondary to trauma or to a preexisting tumor.

Giant cell tumor or osteoclastoma (GCT)

Age: any, but typically 20–35.

Site: metaphyseal with spread through the physeal plate and into the epiphysis, probably arises from within the physeal plate itself.

Bones involved: 50 percent in the knee, but other long bones as well as in the patella, spine, and acetabular roof.

Radiographic appearance: eccentric and expansatile with a gradual transition zone from tumor to normal bone. They may have a soap bubble appearance and may break through the cortex or subchondral bone into the joint (Fig. 7-12).

Treatment: surgery, but 10 percent recur and a few may be premalignant or actually malignant.

Differential diagnosis: aneurysmal bone cyst, fibrocortical defect, chondromyxoid fibroma, plasmocytoma, or osteosarcoma.

Comment: it is not possible to state on radiographic grounds alone if a giant cell tumor is benign or malignant (see illustration). In fact, it is unfortunately also often difficult on histologic grounds to be entirely certain either, and the patient should be carefully watched for evidence of recurrence following surgery.

Now let us turn our attention to leukemia, lymphoma of bone and the plasma cell tumors:

Leukemia

Leukemic involvement of bone is seen in about 50 percent of children with leukemia but is rare in adults. The classic radiographic appearance is that of radiolucent lines in the metaphysis (Fig. 7-13) but periosteal reactions, fractures, lytic areas, and generalized osteopenia may also be seen.

Lymphoma of Bone

Bone changes are seen in about 15 percent of patients with lymphoma. The lesions are usually poorly defined and may be lytic or mixed lytic and blastic which is relatively common (Fig. 7-14). The classical finding is a dense white "ivory" vertebral body which is typically seen in Hodgkin's disease.

Ewing's sarcoma

Age: any, but 80 percent occur before 20.

Symptoms: pain, swelling, fever, anemia, elevated ESR.

Site: central diaphyseal which was actually the classic description but only occurs in 25 percent. More often Ewing's sarcoma is metaphyseal (60 percent) in long bones and it may occur in flat bones.

Bones involved: femur, tibia, fibula, and pelvis.

Radiographic appearance: onion-skin periosteal reaction in long bones with underlying intramedullary destruction (Fig. 7-15A). In the pelvis, reactive new bone formation can occur (Fig. 7-15B).

Treatment: radiotherapy, chemotherapy.

Prognosis: 5-year survival rate is now over 60 percent.

Reticulum cell sarcoma

Age: 20–40.

Site: diaphyseal in femur, humerus, other long bones, clavicle, and ribs.

Symptoms: marked well-being of patient.

Radiographic appearance: permeative destruction of intramedullary cancellous bone and overlying cortical bone with little or no periosteal reaction (Fig. 7-16).

Treatment: surgery, radiotherapy, and chemotherapy.

Prognosis: 5-year survival rate is now over 75 percent.

Multiple myeloma

Myeloma is one of the most important and frequently occurring primary bone tumors. Following a brief description of the classical findings, the different types of plasmacytoma and myeloma variants will be reviewed.

Age: mainly over 50 but may occur earlier.

Sex: males predominate.

Symptoms: bone pain, backache, neurologic signs, weight loss, cachexia, and unexplained osteoporosis.

Site: intramedullary and diaphyseal.

Bones involved: vertebrae 66 percent, ribs 45 percent, skull 40 percent, shoulder girdle 40 percent, pelvis 30 percent, long bones 25 percent.

Radiographic features: sharply defined "punched out" lytic lesions (Fig. 7-17A,B); occasionally expansatile, and seen in association with pathologic fractures and unexplained osteoporosis.

Other features: 60 percent of patients with myeloma have Bence Jones proteinuria, and 95 percent of patients have abnormalities of their plasma proteins.

Comment: unexplained generalized osteoporosis in a young male patient may be caused by multiple myeloma.

Treatment: radiotherapy and chemotherapy.

Prognosis: 5-year survival rate 20 percent.

VARIANTS.

1. *Extramedullary plasmacytoma:* involves the soft tissues of the sinuses or nose and lies outside the scope of this book.
2. *Solitary osseous myeloma (plasmacytoma):* usually presents as an expansatile metaphyseal lesion or occurs in a rib, the acetabular roof or sacrum, and has a lytic soap-bubble appearance. It looks benign and not unlike a giant cell tumor (Fig. 7-17C), but virtually all of the patients with plasmacytomas go on to develop multiple myeloma in due course.

SOME COMMENTS ON MYELOMA.   Many complications occur in association with multiple myeloma, including amyloidosis, renal failure, hypercalcemia, and anemia.

Prior to having an intravenous pyelogram, a patient with multiple myeloma must not be dehydrated otherwise renal failure may ensue due to the precipitation of casts and cells in the renal tubules.

There are a number of methods of differentiating multiple myeloma from metastases:

1. Myeloma may involve the intervertebral discs and the mandible, whereas metastases rarely do so.
2. Metastases often involve the vertebral pedicles whereas myeloma almost never does so.
3. Although both may be associated with a soft-tissue mass, one should think of myeloma if there is a large soft-tissue mass.

METASTASES

Virtually any malignant tumor may send off distant metastases but if some simple statistics are remembered, then the search for a primary lesion in a patient who presents with a metastasis from an unknown site may be simplified. At autopsy, 75 percent of patients with breast cancer have osseous metastases whereas 32 percent of patients with lung cancer and only 10 percent of patients with gastric or rectal carcinoma have skeletal involvement. Classically, lytic metastases come from the lung, kidney, the intestine, and breast (Fig. 7-18A). Breast metastases, however, can turn sclerotic following almost any kind of therapy: mastectomy, radiotherapy, chemotherapy, and even steroid therapy. Blastic (sclerotic) metastases in a male usually come from the prostate, but may come from a bladder cancer which has invaded the prostatic bed, or from a male breast carcinoma (Fig. 7-18B). A solitary lytic expansatile metastasis which looks benign classically comes from kidney or thyroid, but because bronchogenic carcinoma is one of the most common forms of cancer, solitary lytic metastases are also to be seen in this condition. A metastasis in the periphery (hand or foot) often comes from a bronchogenic carcinoma, and a solitary "ivory" vertebra can be seen in prostatic metastatic disease as well as in Hodgkin's disease, Paget's disease, hemangioma of the vertebral body, and in some rare infections.

REFERENCES

Lodwick GS: The Bones & Joints. Chicago, Year Book, 1971

Ranniger K: Encyclopedia of Medical Radiology, Vol. 5. New York, Springer-Verlag, 1977

Spjut HJ, Dorfman HD, Fechner RE, Ackerman LV: Tumors of Bone & Cartilage, Fascicle 5. Washington, D.C., Armed Forces Institute of Pathology, 1971

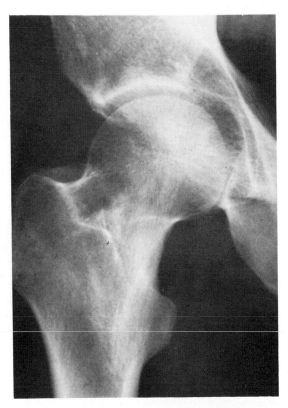

FIGURE 7-1. *Osteoid Osteoma: 39-year-old man.* **A.** Plain film of right hip. This man had complained of pain in his right hip for 18 months and had an operation removing some of the bone from the upper part of the femoral neck. **B.** Tomogram. This film shows a lucent nidus with central sclerosis at the lower end of the femoral calcar (arrow). Note that there is some surrounding sclerosis and a well-defined periosteal reaction proximal to the osteoid osteoma. The lucency and inferiorly placed sclerosis in the upper part of the femoral neck is the site of the previous operation.

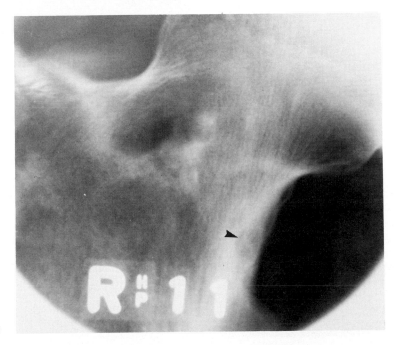

B

FIGURE 7-2. *Typical Osteosarcoma.* **A.** AP. **B.** This 14-year-old boy had a history of pain and swelling over the distal femur for 3 months. The radiographs show a large soft tissue mass with plentiful "sun ray" spiculation representing neoplastic new bone formation. Note the periosteal reaction and Codman's triangles (arrows). The interosseous part of the tumor is difficult to identify but there appears to be patchy sclerosis (particularly laterally) with some lucency. Note that the tumor has respected the physeal plate. (For Figs. 7-2C, D, E, see following pages.)

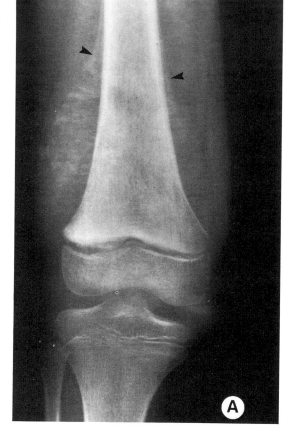

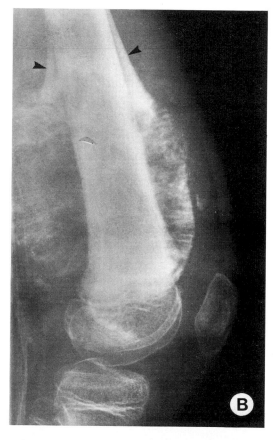

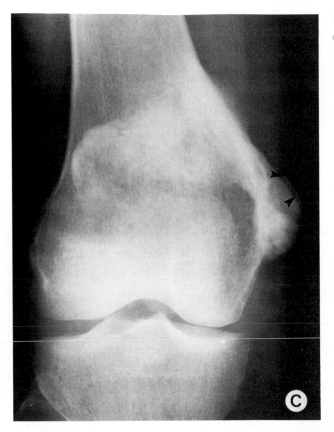

FIGURE 7-2C. *Parosteal Osteosarcoma.* This 31-year-old woman complained of pain in her knee, and this radiograph shows a lobulated extraosseous mass surrounding the distal femur which is associated with a soft-tissue mass and contains a clear-cut lucent line which represents the periosteum (arrows).

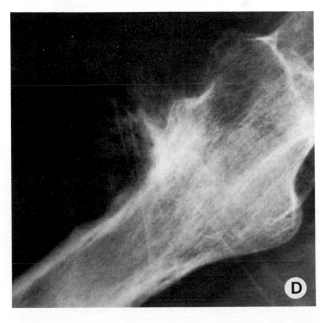

FIGURE 7-2D. *Juxtacortical Osteosarcoma.* This 65-year-old man had pain in his right hip for 6 months prior to having this x-ray. There is a large mass with obvious "sunray" spiculation and erosion of the outer margin of the upper femoral cortex. The endosteal surface of the cortex is somewhat irregular and there is apparent intramedullary spread which was confirmed at biopsy.

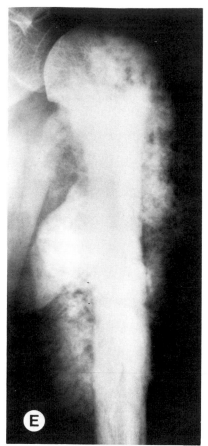

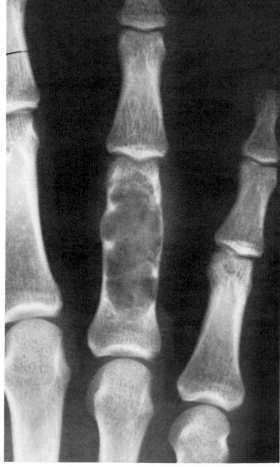

FIGURE 7-2E. *Sarcoma in Paget's Disease.* This elderly male with long-standing Paget's disease developed pain and swelling over his left upper arm. The radiograph shows a multilobulated mass containing dense amorphous neoplastic new bone. On biopsy, this was found to be an osteogenic sarcoma secondary to Paget's disease, and the patient died 3 months later.

FIGURE 7-3. *Enchondroma.* This 25-year-old man presented with pain in his ring finger. The x-ray revealed a well-circumscribed lucency with some expansion of the proximal phalanx, scalloping and thinning of the cortex. The areas of increased density contain amorphous calcification and this lesion has the appearance of a classic enchondroma.

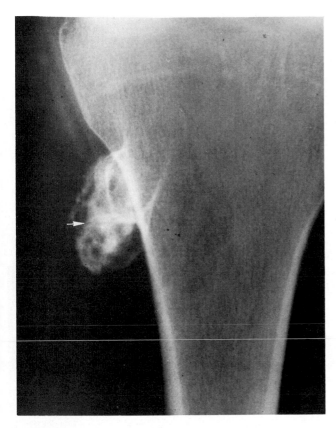

FIGURE 7-4. *Osteochondroma.* This 36-year-old male patient complained of pain in his left knee. X-rays revealed this exostosis with clear-cut osseous margins but with a dense tip containing flocculent calcifications (arrow). This was removed and found to be benign.

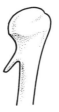 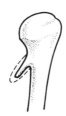 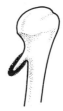

A   Only bone — benign

Bone with uncalcified cartilagenous cap — probably benign

Bone with cartilagenous cap containing flocculent calcification — pre-malignant (8%)

FIGURE 7-5.   **A.** Types of osteochondroma. **B.** Virchow's theory of formation of osteochondromas.

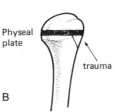 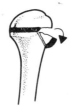 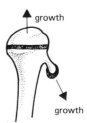

Physeal plate

trauma

growth

growth

B

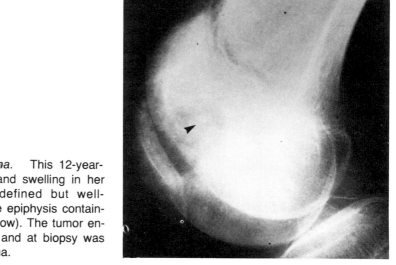

FIGURE 7-6. *Chondroblastoma.* This 12-year-old girl complained of pain and swelling in her knee. There is a poorly defined but well-marginated lucency within the epiphysis containing flocculent calcification (arrow). The tumor encroaches on the joint space and at biopsy was found to be a chondroblastoma.

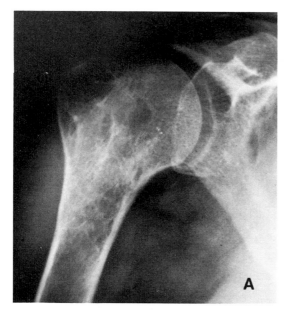

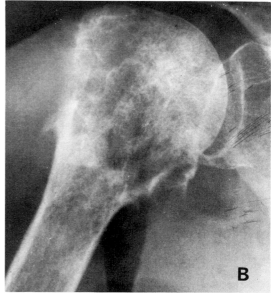

FIGURE 7-7. *Chondrosarcoma: 62-year-old woman.* **A.** Film dated 2/14/69. This patient had had an enchondroma curetted and packed with bone chips 40 years previously. At this time, she was complaining of shoulder pain and the poorly defined lytic areas were thought to be benign and secondary to her previous surgery.

FIGURE 7-7B. Film dated 9/27/71. There is now obvious obstruction of her humeral head with irregular new bone formation in a surrounding soft-tissue mass. At biopsy this was found to be a chondrosarcoma and fits into the description of a "central" secondary type of tumor associated with the presence of benign cartilaginous lesion many years before.

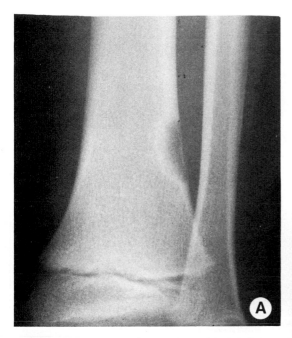

FIGURE 7-8. *Fibrocortical defects: Two Examples.* **A.** Small defect in distal tibia in 10-year-old boy with a peripheral central lucent area roofed in by bone and with a well-defined margin.

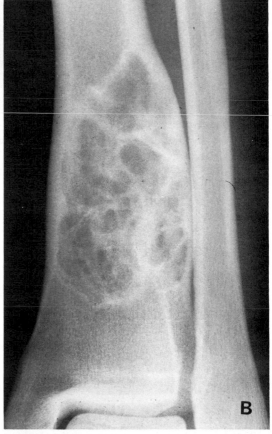

FIGURE 7-8B. Large defect also in the distal tibia of a 20-year-old man who twisted his ankle playing hockey. This one is multilocular and expansatile and "splits" the cortex as well as extends to the other side of the tibia where it has produced new bone formation and buttressing.

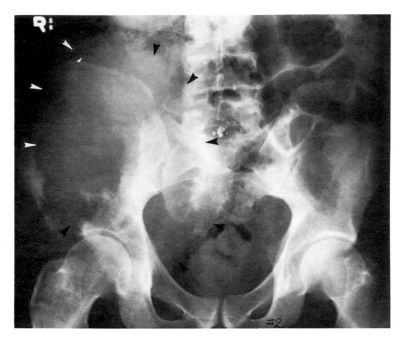

FIGURE 7-9. *Fibrosarcoma.* This 48-year-old man presented with a football sized mass in his lower abdomen (arrows). The x-ray shows massive destruction of the right iliac bone with expansion and has an "explosive" appearance. Note the reactive new bone formation in some of the remaining parts of the pelvis. At biopsy, this was found to be a fibrosarcoma and had already blocked off his right ureter.

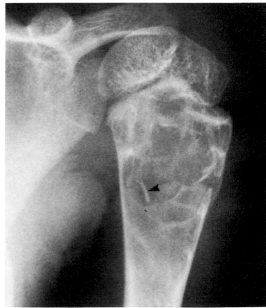

FIGURE 7-10. *Unicameral Bone Cyst.* This 5½-year-old boy came in having had trauma to his left shoulder. There is a large centrally placed expansatile lucency in his upper humerus extending from just below the physeal plate down into the diaphysis where the zone of transition is difficult to see. Note the fracture and the "fallen fragment" (arrow) which represents a small fragment of cortex floating freely within the cyst. These appearances are pathognomonic of a benign bone cyst.

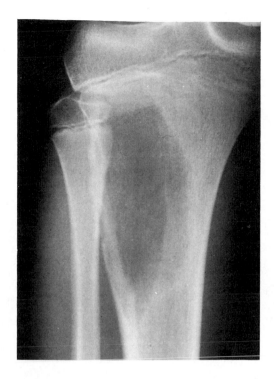

FIGURE 7-11. *Aneurysmal Bone Cyst.* This boy of 14 sustained a blow to his left knee 3 weeks before this film was taken. There is a well-marginated eccentric unilocular expansatile lesion in the metaphysis of his upper tibia. On biopsy, it proved to be an aneurysmal bone cyst and following packing with bone chips; 10 years follow-up has shown no recurrence.

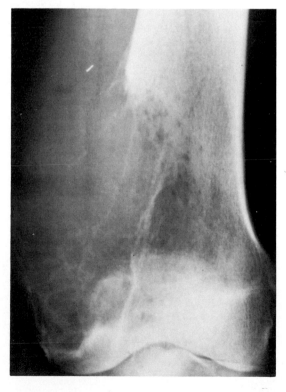

FIGURE 7-12. *Giant Cell Tumor.* This 35-year-old woman presented with pain and swelling on the inner aspect of her left leg for 4 months. The radiograph shows a large eccentric tumor with obvious expansion and soft tissue component. There is no real zone of transition and in fact several small lucencies can be seen in the underlying femur. The tumor contains a few bone trabeculae and spreads from the metaphysis into the epiphysis. Note the Codman's triangle (triangular periosteal reaction) at the proximal end of the lesion. On biopsy this was found to be an extremely benign giant cell tumor in spite of its aggressive-looking radiographic appearance.

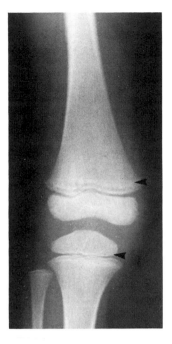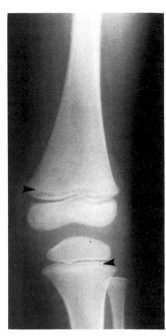

FIGURE 7-13. *Leukemia: Legs.* This 4-year-old child presented with signs of raised intracranial pressure. Radiographs of his long bones show the characteristic findings seen in leukemia: transverse zones of lucency in the metaphysis (arrows) close to the physeal plate.

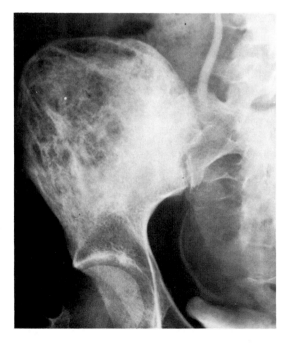

FIGURE 7-14. *Hodgkin's Disease: Pelvis.* There is a mixed sclerotic and lytic lesion in the right iliac bone of this 32-year-old woman who has had Hodgkin's disease for 5 years. At biopsy, this proved to be lymphomatous involvement of bone which is seen in about 15 percent of patients. (Incidentally the IVP was normal.)

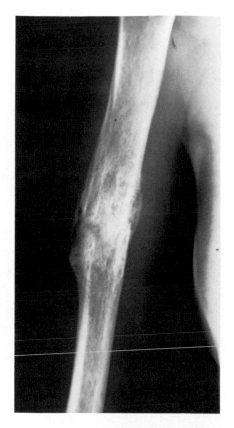

A

FIGURE 7-15. *Ewing's Sarcoma.*   **A.** Humerus. There is a centrally placed permeative destructive lesion involving the medullary canal and cortex and producing a marked periosteal reaction in this 23-year-old girl who was found to have a classic Ewing's sarcoma, which responded well to radiotherapy. **B.** Pelvis. This girl of 19 presented with pain and swelling over her right hip. This radiograph showed a predominantly sclerotic lesion in the right iliac bone associated with a soft tissue mass. At biopsy this was found to be Ewing's sarcoma.

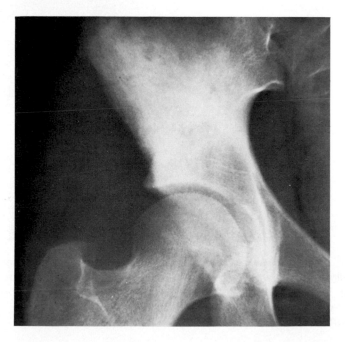

B

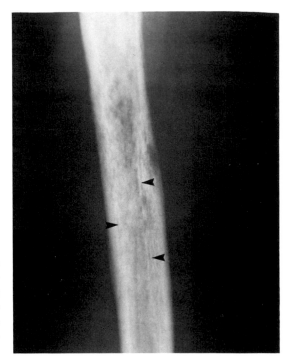

FIGURE 7-16. *Reticulum Cell Sarcoma: Humerus.* There is a permeative diaphyseal lesion involving both cancellous and cortical bone with little periosteal reaction in this 25-year-old female patient. There is also some endosteal new bone formation (arrows) which is indicative of a bone marrow lesion, in this case a reticulum cell sarcoma.

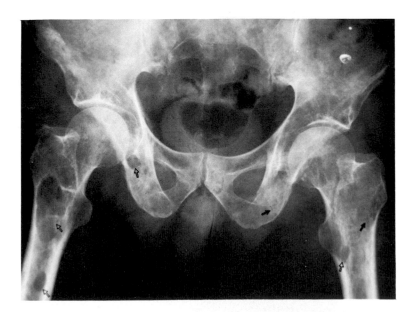

A

FIGURE 7-17. *Multiple Myeloma.*   **A.** Pelvis. This elderly male patient is riddled with well-defined "punched out" lytic areas throughout his pelvis and upper femurs (hollow arrows). The diagnosis of multiple myeloma was made several years previously and he has been on chemotherapy, hence the appearance of new bone formation in a number of areas (solid arrows). (For Figs. 7-17B, C see facing page.)

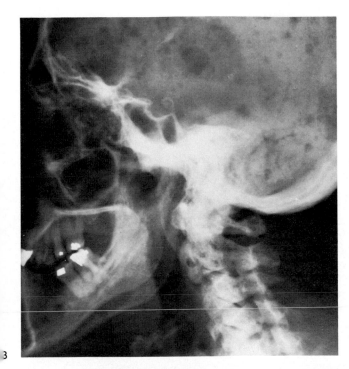

B

FIGURE 7-17B. Skull and cervical spine. There are multiple "punched out" lytic areas in the skull, mandible, and spine of this 72-year-old man with a 12-year history of multiple myeloma. **C. Solitary plasmacytoma.** This 65-year-old man presented with pain in his buttocks. There is a huge multilobular soap-bubble appearing tumor involving the sacrum and right iliac bones. On further work-up this was a solitary lesion, his plasma and urinary proteins were normal and a biopsy revealed a plasmacytoma. Five years after the initial diagnosis was made, the patient developed the classic features of multiple myeloma.

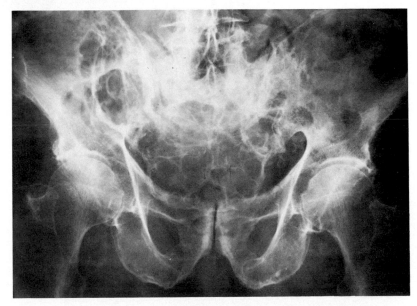

C

FIGURE 7-18. *Metastases.* **A.** Lytic. This 64-year-old woman had breast cancer for 4 years prior to complaining of pain in her right leg. There are multiple lytic areas with a permeative pattern throughout the posterior cortex in association with a periosteal reaction. A radiographic survey showed similar lesions throughout the skeleton. These represent widespread metastases from the primary breast carcinoma. **B.** Blastic. There are multiple areas of increased density throughout the pelvis of this 61-year-old man with prostatic carcinoma. Note that there are several "ivory" vertebrae. There are also some lytic areas and in particular the left pubic ramus has been destroyed. There is a pathologic fracture of the symphysis pubis.

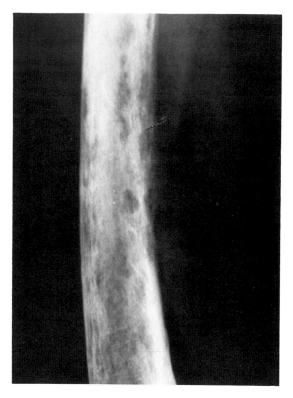

A

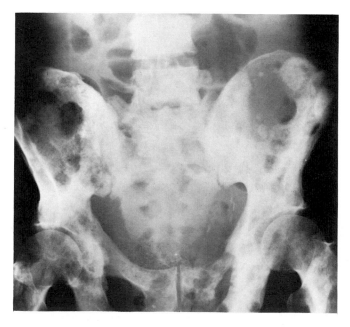

B

EIGHT

Special Procedures

The most frequently used special procedure in the investigation of lesions of the musculoskeletal system is arthrography, which will be discussed in detail. Otherwise fluoroscopy, tomography, magnification, and stereoscopy constitute a group of noninvasive special radiographic techniques related to the skeleton. Radioisotope techniques are extremely useful in the early diagnosis of osteomyelitis and stress fractures but are more routinely used for the investigation of suspected metastatic disease. Angiography has a particular use in the investigation of major trauma and a somewhat less important use with respect to bone tumors. Ultrasound has few indications in the investigation of bone lesions and the CT scanner is only now being evaluated although it appears to have promise in the investigation of major trauma to the hip and shoulder, in the investigation of spinal lesions, to determine the bone mineral content of the vertebral bodies, and also to determine the full extent of tumors. Finally, closed bone biopsies performed by the radiologist are becoming commonplace for the investigation of infections of the spine and solitary tumors in the peripheral skeleton.

ARTHROGRAPHY

Although it is possible theoretically to inject a contrast agent into any articular space in the body (including the temporomandibular joints, interphalangeal joints, and the acromioclavicular joint), the joints that are most commonly investigated are the knee, shoulder, ankle, and wrist. The indications, technique, and appearances vary so that each joint will be considered separately.

The Knee

The most common indication for arthrography of the knee is in patients with suspected meniscal tears, although suspected cruciate and collateral ligament tears, loose bodies, early arthritis, infractions of cartilage, and suspected Baker's cysts are also important indications.

Scout films should be taken as before any special procedure. Knee arthrography involves placing a needle in the joint usually under the patella with a lateral approach and the procedure is performed under fluoroscopic control. About 50 ml of room air (or carbon dioxide) and 4 ml of positive contrast (for example 60 percent Renografin) are used. This is known as a "double contrast" arthrogram, i.e., air mixed with a positive contrast agent. One in 1000 epinephrine solution, 0.5 ml, can be used to delay absorption of the contrast agent from the joint. AP and lateral views of the knee are taken to look for major abnormalities, and then a series of 12 coned-down films are taken of each meniscus from front to back. The films are inspected for meniscal tears (Fig. 8-1), for the appearance of the synovial tent over the cruciates (Fig. 8-2) as well as for evidence of a loose body, cartilage damage, or for a Baker's cyst (Fig. 8-3).

Complications of arthrography are few although a transient synovitis is often seen arthroscopically for the first 2 to 5 days following an arthrogram. The accuracy of knee arthrography should be in the region of 90 percent for medial meniscal tears, and 80 percent for lateral meniscal tears. One should be aware of three main pitfalls: (1) the meniscus should be seen in profile separated from the articular cartilage of both the femur and the tibia (This is known as an "orthograde" view.); (2) there is a small fat pad anteriorly, which may obscure the anterior horn of either meniscus; (3) the tendon of the popliteus muscle actually passes obliquely through the posterior horn of the lateral meniscus, and it is frequently difficult to assess this part of the lateral meniscus without a proper understanding of the normal anatomy.

One final comment is necessary. *Arthroscopy* is also a relatively simple technique for the orthopedist to perform, although it is more painful and time-consuming for the patient. Whereas arthrography is accurate with respect to finding meniscal tears and demonstrating Baker's cysts, arthroscopy is accurate in finding loose bodies, identifying cruciate tears, and is extremely useful for performing minor surgical procedures without resorting to an arthrotomy.

The Shoulder

The indications for arthrography of the shoulder include investigating a frozen shoulder (which is usually caused by fibrosing capsulitis), in identifying loose bodies or tears of the rotator cuff (Fig. 8-4) as well as in examining the shoulder joint in patients with recurrent subluxation. The needle is usually inserted into the shoulder joint anteriorly under fluoroscopic control and either a "double contrast" or a single positive contrast arthrogram may be performed.

The Hip

There are two different groups of indications for performing hip arthrography. On the one hand, hip arthrography is used in patients who have suspected loose bodies (Fig. 8-5), early arthritis, or a suspected infection; on the other hand, arthrography is used in patients with total hip replacements or other prostheses looking for evidence of infection, loosening, or capsular fibrosis (Fig. 8-6).

Other Joints

Although arthrography may be performed on any joint in the body, the most common indications for the investigation of joints other than knee, shoulder, and hip are probably arthrography of the *wrist* (for determining the degree of damage in rheumatoid arthritis); arthrography of the *temporomandibular joint* (in looking for damage to the S-shaped cartilage which occurs in recurrent subluxation); arthrography of the *elbow* (looking for loose bodies); and *discograms* (which are used to investigate the integrity of the intervertebral disc).

FLUOROSCOPY

Although fluoroscopy is an inherent part of arthrography, fluoroscopy is used in many other orthopedic situations, such as in looking at the range of motion of a joint or in attempting to realign the two ends of a fracture. Orthopedic surgeons also routinely use fluoroscopy in the operating room in many pinning and nailing procedures, such as total hip replacements and the realignment of fracture fragments. It is important to remember that it is usual to make some permanent record of the findings at fluoroscopy, and this may be achieved using plain films, cine, videotapes, or taking polaroid pictures.

TOMOGRAPHY

Although some radiologists do not consider tomography to be indicated in musculoskeletal radiography, there are a number of specific uses in which tomography is useful, such as in the investigation of suspected spinal infections, in examining the integrity of the atlantoaxial joint in rheumatoid arthritis (Fig. 6-11), and in looking for evidence of nonunion of a fracture. Tomography can also help delineate the margins and contents of bone tumors in more detail (Fig. 7-1) as well as in certain other situations (Fig. 8-5).

MAGNIFICATION

One of the prime indications for the use of magnification radiography is better delineation of certain entities in the skeleton. Magnification may be "primary" using a microfocal spot tube or "secondary" using a magnifying glass. Uses of magnification include the assessment of early changes in arthritis (particularly rheumatoid) and metabolic bone disease (particularly hyperparathyroidism) as well as in the definition of discrete fractures and early infections, particularly of the extremities.

STEREOSCOPY

This technique has largely dropped out of fashion, but it can still be useful in assessing complex fractures around the hip or shoulder girdle as well as in complex skull and facial injuries. Stereoscopy is achieved by taking a standard radiograph of the area of interest, moving the x-ray tube 6 inches, say in a lateral direction, and taking a second radiograph. If the two radiographs are viewed side by side and either one crosses one's eyes or uses a special prism, a three-dimensional effect can be easily achieved.

NUCLEAR MEDICINE

Bone scans are positive in many of the abnormalities which have been discussed in this book, but there are specific indications for radionuclide studies. For instance, the ideal way to work up a patient with suspected bony metastases is to perform a bone scan initially. If that scan proves to be positive, then it is necessary to radiograph those areas that are positive on the scan to exclude such benign conditions as old fractures, arthritis, or Paget's disease. There are two important indications for the use of radioisotope scans in skeletal radiology, however: (1) in the early diagnosis of osteomyelitis (the scan is positive within 48 hours, whereas the x-rays may not show any abnormality for 10 days); and (2) in the investigation of possible stress fractures, particularly of the tibia where the scan will be positive within 24 to 48 hours, and the x-rays may remain negative for 3 weeks. The most common indication for performing a bone scan is undoubtedly in patients with suspected metastases (Fig. 8-7) in which case the scan will almost always be positive if skeletal metastases are present. The exceptions occur in two situations: (1) in those rare cases where the metastases have become quiescent, which can be seen in breast and prostatic carcinoma following therapy; and (2) in lesions which produce little or no bony reaction such as in multiple myeloma.

ANGIOGRAPHY

One of the indications for angiography in skeletal radiology is in the delineation of the blood supply to the bone tumors. It is often useful to know about the vascularity of a tumor before it is biopsied. Another indication for angiography is in a severely traumatized patient in whom damage to the vessels is suspected (Fig. 8-8). It is a matter of some urgency to perform an arteriogram on patients with major fractures involving the pelvis of long bones because if a major artery is occluded or ruptured, the vessel frequently goes into spasm initially only to dilate several hours or days later, and the patient may exsanguinate.

ULTRASOUND

This has few proven uses in musculoskeletal work although attempts have been made to examine the volume of the spinal canal, the ligamentous architecture of joints (particularly the knee), and to differentiate between solid and cystic tumors of long bones using ultrasound techniques.

CT SCANNING

The place of CT scanning in orthopedic radiology has not yet been fully assessed. Thus far, the CT scanner has proven useful in two main areas: (1) in determining the extent of bone tumors both in and around the bone and outside in the soft tissues (Fig. 8-9) and (2) in the investigation of complex fractures, particularly of the shoulder and hip girdle. Possible future applications of CT scanning in the skeleton are the measurement of bone mineral, the assessment of spinal stenosis, and in looking at the ligamentous integrity of the knee.

BONE BIOPSIES

Biopsies of tumors of the musculoskeletal system may be closed or open. Open (operative) biopsies lie outside the scope of this book. With a trochar, cannula, and a cutting needle (or trephine), it is possible to biopsy both peripheral and spinal lesions under local anesthetic. The indications for closed biopsy include all those lesions which are probably not going to be operated on, i.e., suspected benign bone tumors (particularly of the peripheral bones), suspected infections (often in the spine), and suspected metastatic disease. Various needles are available and the technique is to acquire a core biopsy of the lesion and to send it for a "frozen section." The patient should be sedated and plentiful local anesthetic used, because penetration of the periosteum by the needle can be painful. There are few reported complications, although pneumothoraces can occur in association with rib biopsies, and bleeding occurs following biopsy of aneurysmal bone cysts and vascular metastases, for example, from a hypernephroma.

REFERENCES

Butt WP, McIntyre JL: Double-contrast arthrography of the knee. Radiology 92:487–499, 1969
Freiberger RD, Kaye JJ, Spiller, J: Arthrography. New York, Appleton, 1979
Guilford WB: Shoulder arthrography: a clinical review and practical applications. Appl Radiol 6:133–157, 1977

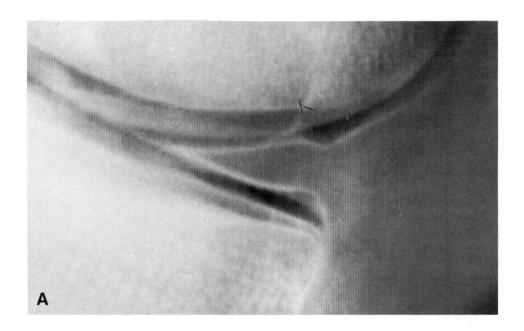

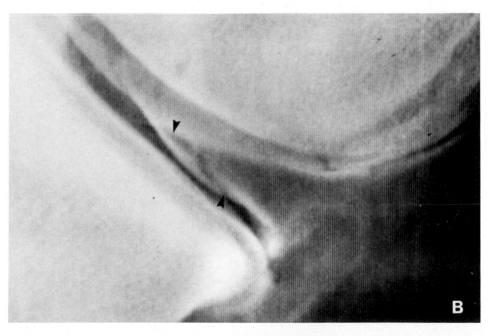

FIGURE 8-1. *Knee Arthrography.*   **A.** Normal. In this coned-down view of the central part of the medial meniscus, the articular surface of the femur and tibia are well seen and the normal meniscus is clearly seen separated from them by air. **B.** Tear. Posterior horn medial meniscus. This 17-year-old boy twisted his knee. Arthrography shows a tear of the medial meniscus (arrows).

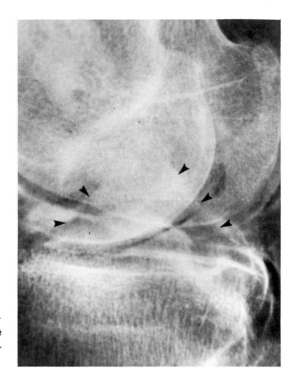

FIGURE 8-2. *Knee Arthrography: Normal Cruciates.* In this slightly oblique lateral view, the "tent" of synovium which lies over the cruciate ligaments can be clearly seen (arrows).

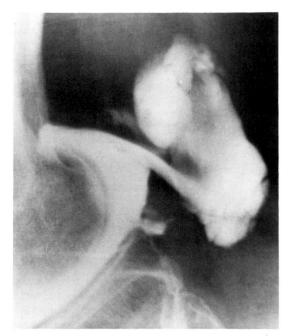

FIGURE 8-3. *Baker's or Popliteal Cyst.* In this single contrast knee arthrogram, there is an obvious communication between the knee joint itself and a large posteriorly lying cyst which actually represents the semi-membranosa-gastrocnemius bursa.

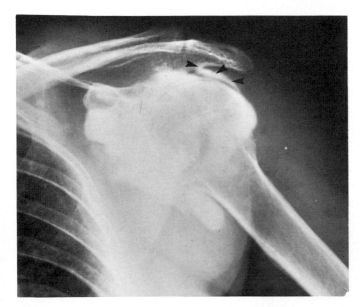

FIGURE 8-4. *Shoulder Arthrography: Tear of Rotator Cuff.* There is a capacious shoulder joint in this 54-year-old patient with pain and difficulty in motion of his left shoulder. On arthrography, contrast can be seen running through the rotator cuff (arrows) and into the subdeltoid bursa.

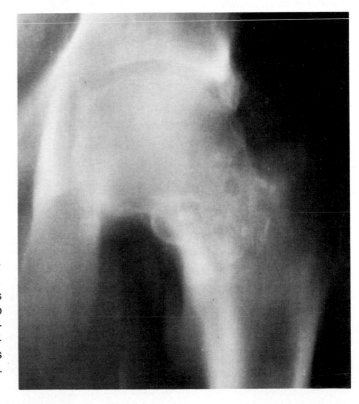

FIGURE 8-5. *Hip Arthrography: Synovial Osteochondromatosis.* **A.** Tomogram of the left hip. This 49-year-old man had pain in his hip for 3 years. Plain films and tomography showed many areas of calcification plus possible loose bodies around the femoral neck. (For Fig. 8-5B see following page.)

A

163

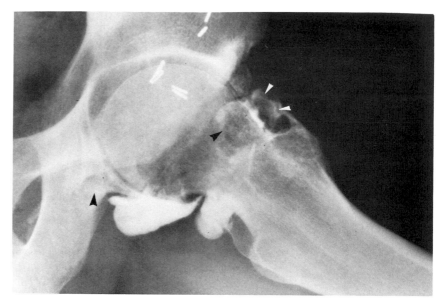

B

FIGURE 8-5B. Arthrography revealed a rather
small joint capsule as well as multiple loose bodies
(arrows). These appearances are characteristic of
synovial osteochondromatosis.

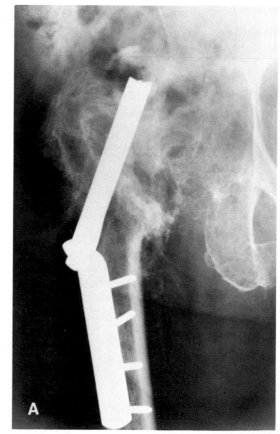

A

FIGURE 8-6. *Hip Arthrography: Infected Pin and
Plate.* This 85-year-old woman had fallen and
sustained an intratrochanteric fracture of her right
femur 3 years before, which had been treated by
internal fixation with a fixed pin and plate. She was
admitted complaining of pain in the hip. **A.** Plain
film. This reveals loss of the femoral head, subluxation of the upper femur laterally, and a lucency
surrounding the pin itself. (For Fig. 8-6B see facing
page.)

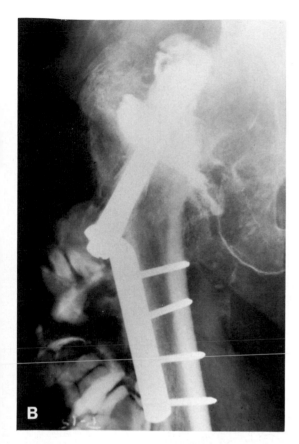

FIGURE 8-6B. Hip arthrogram. On arthrography, contrast went around the pin and out laterally into a huge and infected bursa lying in the muscles of the thigh.

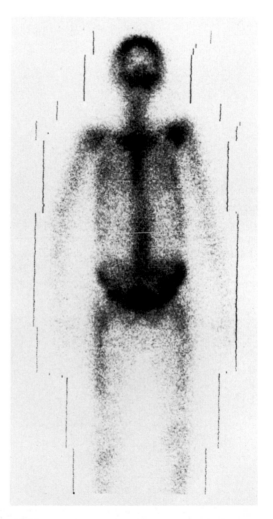

FIGURE 8-7. *Bone Scan: Metastases.* This 58-year-old man had a presumptive diagnosis of Paget's disease, and a bone scan showed multiple areas of increased uptake (the skull, left shoulder, and left iliac bone). His alkaline phosphatase was slightly elevated but his acid phosphatase was extremely high and biopsy of the left scapula and iliac bone showed metastatic deposits from a prostatic carcinoma.

FIGURE 8-8. *Angiography.* This young man fell off his motorcycle at high speed. He sustained injuries to his skull, pelvis, and left leg. There were no pulses below the knee in the leg and a femoral arteriogram was performed which showed rupture of the popliteal artery just below the knee (arrow).

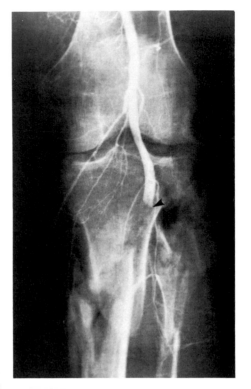

FIGURE 8-9. *CT Scan: L4 Level.* This 52-year-old man was presented with back pain and a lytic lesion of L4. This cut from a CT scan showed destruction of the vertebral body as well as the posterior elements on the left and a huge soft tissue mass. On biopsy, this was found to be multiple myeloma.

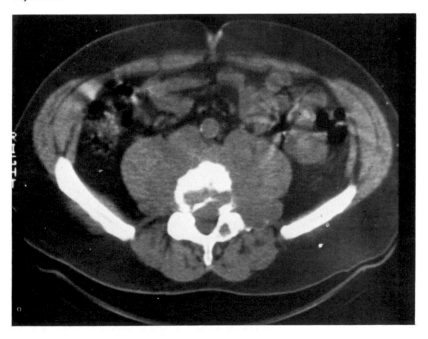

NINE

Other Conditions of Interest

It appears that in most books on bone disease a number of conditions seem to be largely ignored. This chapter is an attempt to redress this deficiency. Five largely unrelated conditions will be discussed, the first of which is common and is a systemic condition. This is followed by a brief description of the bone manifestations of another systemic disease which in turn is followed by short comments on three hematologic diseases, each of which affect the skeleton in a specific way.

Diabetes

The classic musculoskeletal complications of diabetes involve the foot and are known as *diabetic osteo-(arthro)-pathy*. This is a curious mixture of bone resorption and bone formation and has a very characteristic appearance (Fig. 9-1). There is *resorption* around many of the MTP joints with loss of the *metatarsal heads* as well as dissolution of one or more phalanges. The whole process is probably due to small vessel disease and can be associated with cellulitis or even *frank osteomyelitis*, often on the ball of the foot. More proximally, a *periosteal reaction* may be seen surrounding the proximal ends of the metatarsals. This may occur de novo but may be associated with *neuropathic joints* at the tarsometatarsal or metatarsophalangeal levels. Occasionally, neuropathic (Charcot's) joints can be seen elsewhere in diabetes (particularly in the ankles) (see Chap. 6). Diabetics are more prone to get *infections* both in the soft tissue and skeleton as well as having an increased susceptibility to septic arthritis. Finally, it should be remembered that medial wall arterial calcification (*Mönckebergs sclerosis*) is seen in the periphery of many diabetics.

Sarcoidosis

Although sarcoidosis classically involves the chest presenting with hilar adenopathy ultimately going onto interstitial pulmonary fibrosis, it is said that 4 percent of patients with intrathoracic sarcoid have characteristic bone changes. In my opinion, however, osseous sarcoid is rarer than this, although since skeletal involvement is usually asymptomatic it is difficult to be certain of the true incidence. The appearances are very characteristic with well-defined lucencies occurring in the phalanges classically at the distal ends of the middle phalanx (Fig. 9-2). Note that the lesion spreads from the diaphysis through the metaphysis and into the epiphysis often affecting the distal interphalangeal joint. Osseous sarcoid has been described elsewhere in the skeleton, including involvement of the right saroiliac joint similar to that seen in tuberculosis, and is indistinguishable radiographically from a chronic osteomyelitis or bone abscess.

Hemophilia

Musculoskeletal problems should not occur in carefully controlled hemophiliacs. There are, however, four classic skeletal changes described as a result of recurrent bleeding into bones or joints. (1) In young children bleeding into an actual bone produces a cystlike lesion known as a *hemophiliac pseudotumor*. (2) Bleeding into the region of the physeal plate produces *widening* both of the metaphysis and epiphysis as well as characteristic *coarsening* of the trabecular pattern and premature closure of the plate. (3) Recurrent bleeding into a joint itself has two effects and produces a synovitis with hypertrophy of the synovium leading to erosions and irregularities of the joint surfaces (Fig. 6-6) as well as *widening of the intercondylar notch,* which may also be seen in rheumatoid arthritis, tuberculosis, and villonodular synovitis. (4) As a result of blood remaining in the joint, hyaluronidase is released which actually *destroys the articular cartilage* leading to premature osteoarthritis.

Sickle Cell Anemia

Although the majority of patients with sickle cell anemia have some skeletal manifestations of their disease, some patients with sickle cell trait and sickle cell thalassemia also may show the distinctive changes associated with true sickle cell anemia. Anoxia leads to "sickling" of the abnormal red cells which in turn produces infarction. In the skeleton, sickle cell anemia is associated with four characteristic signs (Fig. 9-3A): (1) dense sclerotic areas of intramedullary and cancellous bone infarction; (2) endosteal new bone formation; (3) avascular necrosis, particularly of the femoral head; and (4) a characteristic squaring off of the vertebral end plates into an "H shape" (Fig. 9-3B), which is caused by central infarction with the integrity of the apophyses being maintained by a good secondary blood supply. Also remember (as was mentioned in Chapter 4) that people with sickle cell anemia are more prone to develop infections and although the staphylococcus is still the most common organism involved, salmonella infections are not uncommon in patients with sickle cell anemia.

Thalassemia

Any bone marrow dyscrasia can lead to alterations in the trabecular pattern, particularly in young children. The radiographic appearance of thalassemia includes a hair-on-end skull and widening of the small bones of the hands and feet with a curious fragile, irregular trabecular structure (Fig. 9-4).

Other Lesions

Four more generalized situations that are difficult to classify under any one heading will be presented. The osteochondritides, which may involve virtually every epiphysis in the body, will be followed by a brief discussion on pathologic processes related specifically to the hip joint because this encompasses congenital and traumatic lesions, metabolic bone disease, and the arthritides. Finally, a brief discussion will follow on periosteal reactions and hypertrophic pulmonary osteoarthropathy.

Osteochondritis

This is a large group of conditions involving predominantly overweight male children between the ages of 5 and 11. At least 80 separate types have been described, most of which have eponyms. All of them, however, have a common pathogenesis which is that part of the epiphysis of a bone (if not the whole bone) undergoes avascular necrosis. The reason for this is not properly understood but there seem to be two distinct varieties of osteochondritis: (1) *osteochondritis dissecans* (meaning "dissected or separated") is common, and although it may involve any joint, osteochondritis dissecans is particularly common in the knee where it occurs classically on the lateral aspect of the medial epicondyle (LAME) (Fig. 9-5). The area involved by avascular necrosis may remain in its normal anatomic position surrounded by living bone and inside the cover of the still intact articular cartilage, or may separate from the living bone. Because of continued stress, infraction of the overlying cartilage occurs and the dead bone falls into the joint and thus becomes a loose body (Fig. 9-6). (2) *Osteochondritis* may involve almost any epiphysis or apophysis in the body. The more commonly described ones involve the femoral capital epiphysis (Legg–Calvé–Perthe's disease), the talus (Köhler's disease), the capitulum (Panner's disease), the head of the second metatarsal (Freiberg's disease), the tibial tubercle (Osgood–Schlatter's disease), the insertion of the Achilles tendon into the os calcis (Sinding–Larsen's disease), the lunate (Kienböck's disease), and so on (Fig. 9-7). A third form of osteochondritis was described but this is now thought to have a different etiology. (3) Scheuermann's disease involves the ring-shaped vertebral apophyses above and below each vertebral body (Fig. 9-8A). It has recently been shown that Scheuermann's disease is *not* due to avascular necrosis at all and is in fact probably due to weakness in the vertebral end plates and herniation of disc material between the apophysis and the vertebral body itself. It is thus similar to the etiology of Schmorl's nodes (Fig. 9-8B) and is presumably related to this common condition.

Specific Lesions of the Hip

If we exclude the basic groups of arthritides, tumors, and infections, we are left with a number of conditions that specifically involve the hip joint: one is congenital in origin, one is an osteochondritis, and three are of unknown etiology (Table 9-1).

CONGENITAL DISLOCATION OF THE HIP (CDH).   This is usually associated with a hip dysplasia and many people now refer to the condition as congenital hip dysplasia (CHD). CDH starts at or before birth and if the femoral head does not sit properly within the acetabular labrum, then "congenital dislocation of the hip" develops. It appears that for the correct development of both the acetabulum and the femoral head it is necessary for them to be congruous the majority of the time in early life. The acetabulum has a higher angle than normal and is shallow, whereas the femoral head becomes malformed and subluxes laterally (Fig. 9-9).

LEGG–CALVÉ–PERTHE'S DISEASE.   This is an osteochondritis of the femoral capital epiphysis usually involving somewhat overweight children aged between 4 and 8. Initially it causes flattening and fragmenta-

Table 9-1

A Radiologic Approach to Anomalies Involving the Hip Joint

	CDH	LPD	SCFE	Coxa Valga/Coxa Vara
Acetabulum	Abnormal	—*	—*	—*
Femoral head	Malformed	Often flattened	Slips postero-medially and appears flattened	Normal
Metaphysis	Widened	Widened	Normal	Normal
Neck/shaft angle	Normal	Normal	Normal	Abnormal

Secondary osteoarthritis in later life.

tion of the femoral head which in turn leads to widening of the metaphysis (Fig. 9-8). It results in distortion of the femoral head and although the acetabulum may remain normal, secondary degenerative arthritis often supervenes in later life (Fig. 9-10). Legg–Calvé–Perthe's disease is bilateral in about 25 percent of patients.

SLIPPED CAPITAL FEMORAL EPIPHYSIS (SCFE).   This occurs more frequently in overweight boys aged from 10 to 14, and the etiology is unknown. The head slips posteriorly and somewhat medially. If uncorrected, SCFE also leads to premature degenerative arthritis in the involved hip (Fig. 9-11). It is commonly seen in a minor form where the head slips, yet the acetabulum remains normal.

COXA VARA AND COXA VALGA.   The normal angle between the femoral neck and femoral shaft is 135°. If there are acquired or congenital abnormalities of this angle (valga being greater than 140° and vara being less than 130°), they may lead to pain, premature degenerative arthritis, or to recurrent subluxation.

Periosteal Reaction

Periosteal reaction is commonly seen in osteomyelitis, as callus in fractures and in tumors. There are, however, a number of other conditions in which generalized or localized periosteal reactions occur (Table 9-2). The most common cause of a localized periosteal reaction is varicose veins or a varicose ulcer (Fig. 9-12), whereas probably the most frequent type of generalized periosteal reaction seen is hypertrophic (pulmonary) osteoarthropathy which is discussed below. One final comment about periosteal reactions is relevant, note that abnormal "cotton wool" callus occurs in Cushing's disease, steroid therapy, osteogenesis imperfecta, and with poor immobilization, such as is seen in paralyzed patients.

Table 9-2

Causes of Periosteal Reaction

Generalized	Localized
Vitamin D intoxication	Callus in fractures*
Scurvy	Varicose veins (most common cause of localized periosteal reaction in the legs)
Malnutrition	
Hypertrophic (pulmonary) osteoar-thropathy (see Table 9-3)	Early osteomyelitis
	Myositis ossificans
	(Sub)periosteal trauma
	Osteogenic sarcoma
	Parosteal osteosarcoma
	Metastases
	Other tumors particularly Ewing's sarcoma
	Thyroid acropachy

Most common cause.

Hypertrophic (Pulmonary) Osteoarthropathy

This form of periosteal reaction was first described in association with pulmonary diseases, however, it has become apparent that it occurs in many conditions below the diaphragm, hence hypertrophic osteoar-thropathy is a better term to describe it (Table 9-3). The etiology is unknown, and the patient presents with clubbing, complaining of pain, swelling, and stiffness in the wrist, ankles, or other joints. A diffuse periosteal reaction which is localized usually to the metaphyseal regions of the involved bones is the classic radiographic appearance of hyper-trophic osteoarthropathy (Fig. 9-13).

Table 9-3

Etiology of Hypertrophic (Pulmonary) Osteoarthropathy

Lungs	Abdomen
Bronchogenic carcinoma	Chronic ulcerative colitis, regional enteritis, cholecystitis
Other malignancies: mesothelioma, metastases, squamous cell carcinoma	Pancreatitis, hepatitis, cirrhosis
Chronic bronchitis and bronchiectasis	Gallstones and gallbladder disease
Empyema	Mucoid-producing carcinomas of the stomach and colon
Tuberculosis, sarcoid, fungal infection	
Some congenital heart diseases and left-to-right shunts	
Subacute bacterial endocarditis	
Chronic pericarditis	

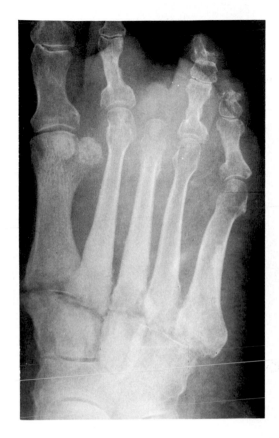

FIGURE 9-1. *Diabetic Osteopathy: Foot.* This 49-year-old man had juvenile onset diabetes. Apart from the amputation of the third toe, there is dissolution of the second and third metatarsal heads, a periosteal reaction around the third metatarsal, and generalized increased density in the second and third metatarsals. Note that there are also destructive changes in many of the tarsometatarsal joints which is indicative of a neuropathic joint. Also medial wall arterial calcification is faintly visible between the second, third as well as the fourth and fifth metatarsals.

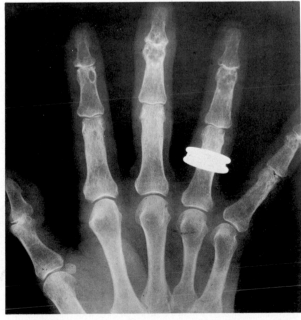

FIGURE 9-2. *Sarcoid: Hand.* There are multilocular lacelike cystic changes in the distal ends of many of the middle phalanges. These are metaphyseal and extend one way into the epiphysis distorting the distal interphalangeal joint and into the diaphysis the other way. All these changes are typical of osseous involvement in sarcoidosis.

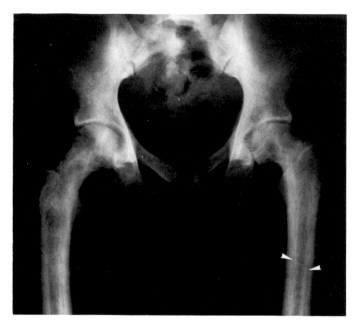

A

FIGURE 9-3. *Sickle Cell Anemia.* **A.** Pelvis. This 24-year-old black male with severe sickle cell anemia shows the characteristic patchy areas of sclerosis representing infarcts in the pelvis and femur. Some of these are large (left iliac bone) and some are tiny (intertrochanteric region of the right femur). Endosteal new bone formation can be clearly seen in both femurs (arrows) and there is avascular necrosis of the left femoral head. **B.** Spine. The characteristic notches can be seen in the end plates of all the thoracic vertebral bodies (arrows) producing the so-called H-shaped vertebra.

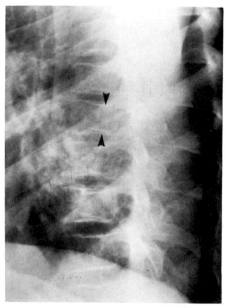

B

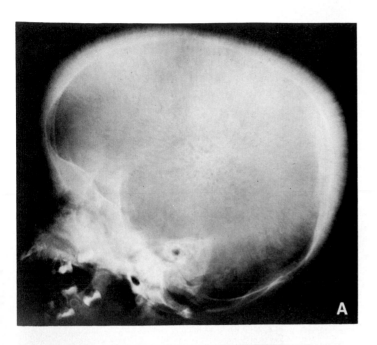

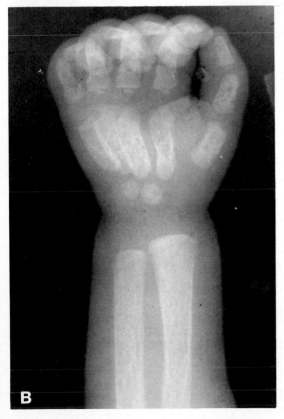

FIGURE 9-4. *Thalassemia.* **A.** Skull. This lateral view shows the characteristic "hair-on-end" appearance seen in many of the hemoglobinopathies. **B.** Hand. This radiograph of the same child shows the abnormal lacelike trabecular pattern seen in thalassemia.

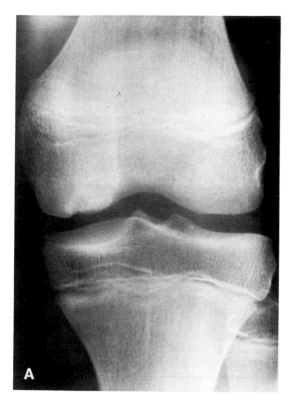

FIGURE 9-5. *Osteochondritis Dissecans: Knee.* **A.** Straight AP view. **B.** Tunnel view. These demonstrate a defect apparently containing a separated fragment (arrow) in this 14-year-old boy with pain in his knee.

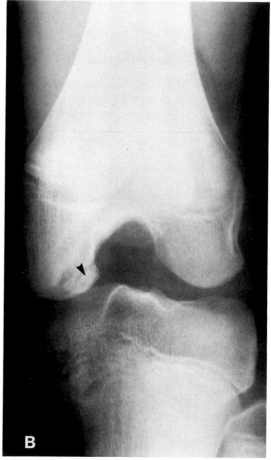

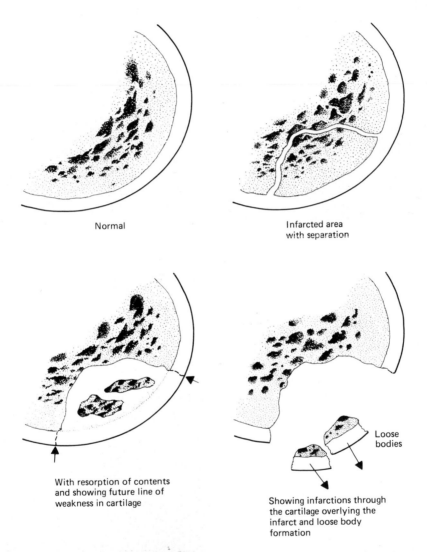

Normal

Infarcted area
with separation

With resorption of contents
and showing future line of
weakness in cartilage

Loose
bodies

Showing infarctions through
the cartilage overlying the
infarct and loose body
formation

FIGURE 9-6. Osteochondritis dissecans: drawings of the stages and outcome of the condition.

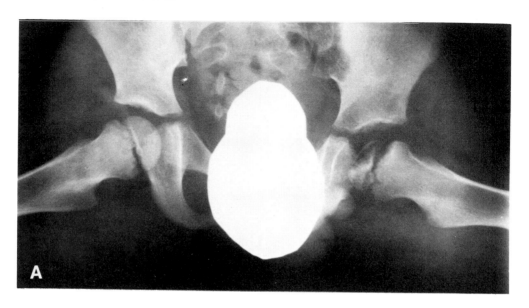

FIGURE 9-7. *Osteochondritis.*   A. Femoral capital epiphysis. (Legg–Calvé–Perthe's disease).
This 13-year-old boy has complained of pain in his
left hip for 2 years. The femoral head on the left is
flattened and disintegrating with areas of increased lucency and sclerosis in association with
irregularity of the physeal plate and widening of
the metaphysis. B. Lunate (Kienböck's disease).
There is obvious increase in density with collapse
and fragmentation of the lunate in this middle-
aged female patient complaining of pain in her
wrist following minor trauma.

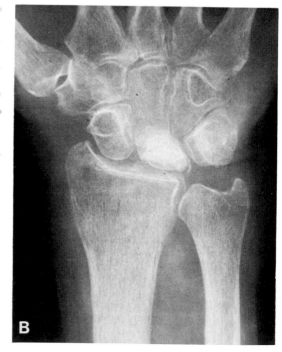

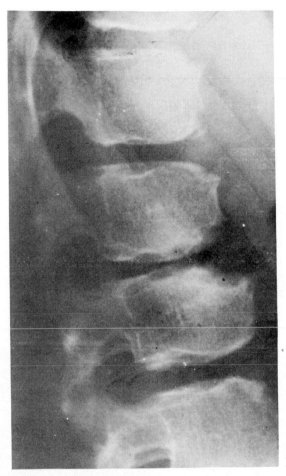

A

FIGURE 9-8. *Vertebral Edge Separation
(Scheuermann's disease).* **A.** Many of the anterior vertebral apophyses are missing and the
underlying bone is apparently eroded and sclerotic. These changes were thought to be typical of
Scheuermann's disease but more recently it has
been shown that there is no evidence of avascular
necrosis or "osteochondritis."

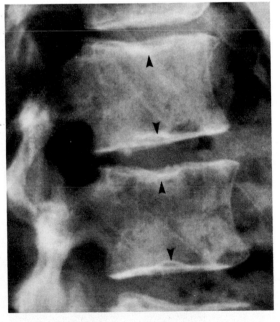

B

FIGURE 9-8B. *Schmorl's Nodes.* A number of
discrete defects can be seen in the end plates of
these vertebral bodies (arrows). These represent
Schmorl's nodes or minor herniations of the disc
through the vertebral end plate.

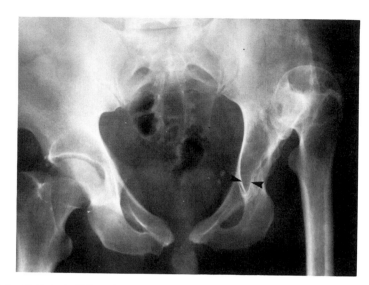

FIGURE 9-9. *Congenital Hip Dysplasia or Congenital Dislocation of the Hip.*   This 37-year-old man presents with a long history of left hip pain and shortening of the left leg. His left acetabulum is almost nonexistent with a wide "tear drop" (arrows) characteristic of a congenital dislocation of the hip. The femoral head is subluxed up and outwards, and there is distortion and degenerative changes of the upper femur with an abnormally large femoral head and foreshortened neck. The right hip is normal.

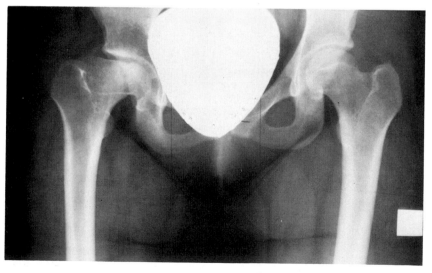

FIGURE 9-10. *Old Legg–Calvé–Perthe's Disease.*   There is flattening and distortion of the right capital femoral epiphysis in this 18-year-old girl complaining of hip pain for 7 years. The head is "mushroomed" and the neck widened, but the acetabulum and tear drop are normal in size, shape, and position.

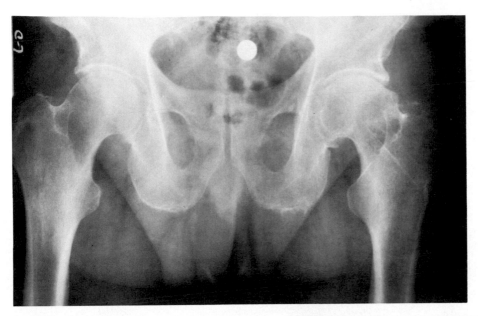

FIGURE 9-11. *Slipped Capital Femoral Epiphysis (SCFE).* This 46-year-old man complained of pain in his left hip during adolescence and a slipped capital femoral epiphysis was diagnosed and treated by using a pin, the tracks of which can still be seen. The head remains slipped medially and downward, however, compare the left side with the right side which also demonstrates a slight slip.

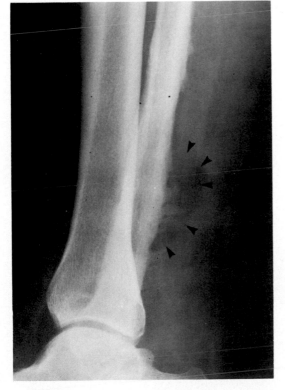

FIGURE 9-12. *Periosteal Reaction in Varicose Veins: Fibula.* There is an irregular, rather jagged periosteal reaction running up the fibula in this 73-year-old woman with a long history of varicose veins. A large area of increased lucency representing a varicose ulcer can be faintly seen (arrows) at the place where the periosteal reaction is at its most marked. At the time this film was taken, the patient had no evidence of infection.

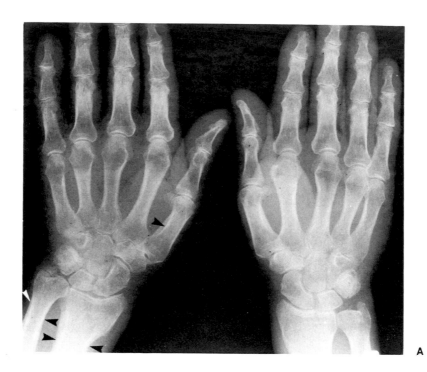

FIGURE 9-13. *Hypertrophic Osteoarthropathy.* **A.** Hands. This 48-year-old smoker presented with pain in his wrists and ankles as well as clubbing of his fingers. Radiographs revealed a marked periosteal reaction around his distal radii and ulnas as well as first metacarpals (arrows). **B.** Chest. The chest x-ray revealed a large mass in the left hilum with a cavitating peripheral pneumonia. At thoracotomy, this proved to be an inoperable bronchogenic carcinoma.

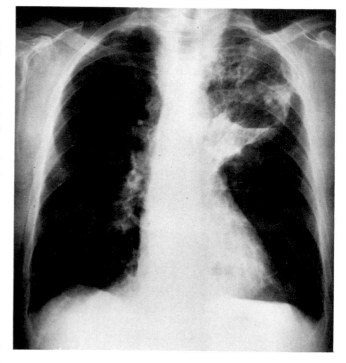

Index

(Italicized numbers refer to tables and figures.)